Mediterranean Diet Cookbook

The complete guide on the Mediterranean diet, with indications, tables and more than 150 recipes to perform

Maggy P. Sert

Copyright © 2020 Maggy P. Sert

All rights reserved.

CONTENTS

PART 1 – THE MEDITERRANEAN DIET 1
1.1 WHAT IS A MEDITERRANEAN DIET? 1
1.2 WHAT ARE THE BENEFITS OF A MEDITERRANEAN DIET? . 4
1.3 THE MEDITERRANEAN DIET PYRAMID 9
1.4 THE MEAL PLAN 13
PART 2 – MEDITERRANEAN DIET RECIPES 15
2.1 LOAVES 15
2.2 BREAKFAST MEALS 36
2.3 MEDITERRANEAN DIET SALADS 65
2.4 MEDITERRANEAN DIET SOUPS 108
2.5 MEDITERRANEAN DIETMAIN DISHES 136
2.6 PIZZAS 194
2.7 DESSERTS, DRINKS AND SMOOTHIES 208
2.8 SNACKS 237
2.9 VEGETARIAN MEDITERRANEAN MEALS 255
PART 3 – CALORIES TABLE 267
3.1 MAIN FOODS 268
3.2 DAIRY 269
3.3 FRESH FRUIT 269
3.3 VEGETABLES 270

MEDITERRANEAN DIET COOKBOOK

PART 1 – THE MEDITERRANEAN DIET

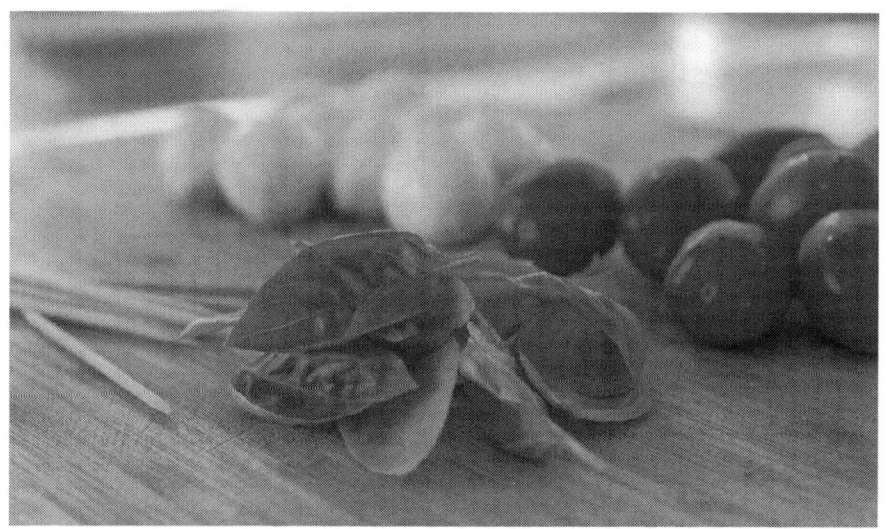

1.1 WHAT IS A MEDITERRANEAN DIET?

A Mediterranean diet is a diet or eating habit observed by people who live in areas close to the Mediterranean Sea. The Mediterranean eating regimen is supplied with a boundless arrangement of new, solid, normal, and healthy nourishments from all nutrition classes. In spite of the fact that there is a more prominent spotlight on specific fixings, no common fixings are avoided. It is one of the most healthy diets in the world as it provides its consumers with healthy nutrition.

BRIEF HISTORY

This diet is known to have originated from the eating habits of people from Crete, Greece, and even Italy in the 20th Century. In view of their mild atmosphere and area, occasional new organic products, vegetables, and fish are common to this region. This heart-sound eating regimen has its inceptions in the Mediterranean basin, generally alluded to as "The Cradle of Society" in light of the fact that the entire history of the antiquated world occurred inside its topographical outskirts.

The genuine inceptions of the Mediterranean eating routine are, be that as it may, lost in time. We may think back to the dietary patterns and examples of the Middle Ages, or much further, to the Roman culture (which displayed the Greek culture) and their distinguishing proof of red wine, bread, and oil as images of their country culture. Numerous individuals in the Mediterranean locale cultivated the land and created organic products; what's more, vegetables; they additionally looked for food.

Meat and dairy were not exceptionally normal in this district, as the atmosphere isn't perfect for touching. Fish, goats, and sheep were the most well-known protein sources.

Its discovery was prior to the results of research conducted in Italy. Ankel Keys, an American scientist discovered that people in specific areas of Italy were less prone to the risk of heart disease, which was eventually traced to their diet. After its publicity by the American scientist in 1975, the Mediterranean diet was still not really heard of, neither was it accepted by people of other nations.

Since this diet started gaining recognition in the 1990s, everybody has been discussing the Mediterranean eating regimen; however, just a bunch of individuals tail it appropriately. For a few, the Mediterranean eating routine is about pizza, and for other people, it's pasta and meat sauce.

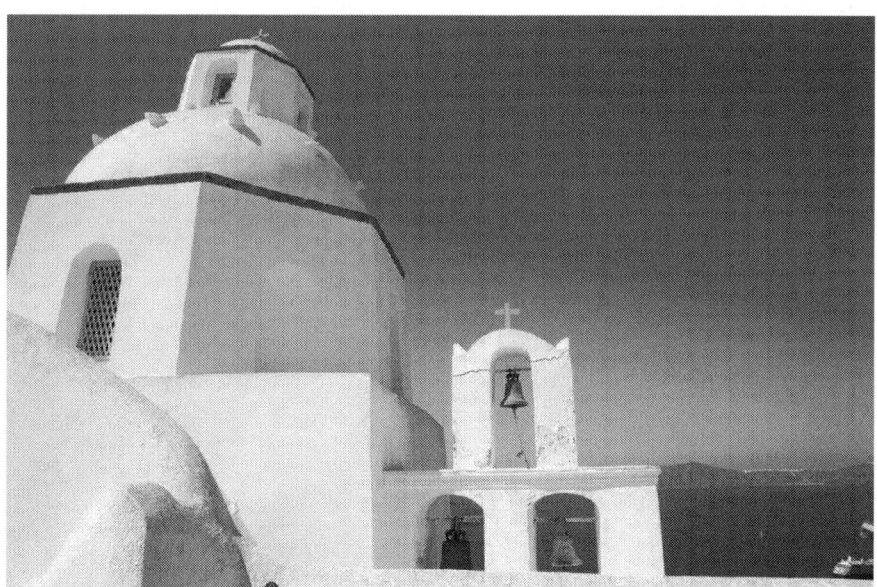

1.2 WHAT ARE THE BENEFITS OF A MEDITERRANEAN DIET?

The significance of eating a clean and even eating routine for improved wellbeing and better personal satisfaction is understood by most of us; however, not many of us really put this into training.

While some spend more time engrossed in our daily activities, we will, in general, choose quick and simple choices with regards to the food we eat. Unconsciously, we have adopted frozen meals, fast food, and food with handled nourishments as our first alternatives. Apart from the generally known fact that this diet reduces your risk of heart disease, it also provides other health benefits.

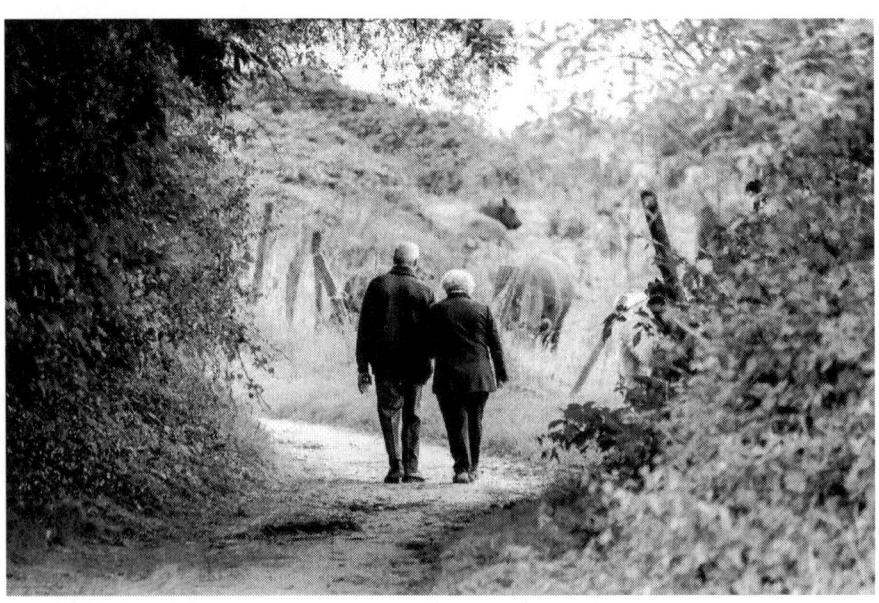

The Mediterranean diet also reduces the risk of cancer, diabetes, and depression. It is proficient in reducing the weight of obese persons and increasing one's cognitive ability. It is also believed that strict adherence to this diet increases the length of one's telomeres.

DIETARY COMPONENTS OF THE MEDITERRANEAN DIET

This diet is based on the consumption of healthy fats from olive oil, olives, avocado, fatty seafood, nuts and seeds, Legumes, Fruits, Vegetables, and Whole grains. Depending on the consumer, adjustments can be made, while noting that seafood should be moderately consumed and the consumption of red meat should be limited.

Depending on the consumer, the meal plan may differ, but the composition of each food group must be in accordance with the Mediterranean diet's plan.

A FEW THINGS TO KNOW TO GET YOU STARTED ON THE MEDITERRANEAN DIET

If you have decided to embark on this journey or you already have, here are a few tips to help you through.

- One most important tip is to take it one step at a time and never give up.

- Always have a meal plan and try as much as possible to stick to the plan. If you don't, well….. keep at it!

- Have breakfast each day, regardless of how bustling your timetable

At this point, you realize that the morning meal is your most significant dinner of the day. A supplement rich breakfast—stuffed with organic products, vegetables, entire grains, furthermore, other fiber-rich nourishments—will help your vitality levels for the afternoon and keep you full until your next feast.

- Know the contrast among sound and unfortunate fats

Monounsaturated fats are solid fats found in olives, sunflower seeds, avocados, additional virgin olive oil, and nuts.

Polyunsaturated oils, additionally solid fats, are found in soybean, sunflower, corn, what's more, safflower oils.

These advance heart wellbeing and, furthermore, lower terrible cholesterol levels. Immersed fats and trans fats, then again, are viewed as unfortunate fats, what's more, over-utilization can expand your danger of cardiovascular diseases and furthermore raise your terrible cholesterol levels.

- Eat, however many vegetables as could be expected under the circumstances in each supper. Vegetables are wealthy in fiber, which helps keep you full more, and furthermore supports absorption. Burden up your sandwiches, soups, omelets, stews, pizza, and some other supper with new vegetables, herbs, and flavors.

- Diminish your meat consumption.

By lessening your red meat admission, you will likewise be decreasing your admission of soaked and trans fats found in meat items. You can every so often have red meat; however, it ought to be in little bits and from lean cuts.

- Seafood consumption at least twice a week

Fish, for example, salmon, fish, sardines, and herring, are wealthy in omega-3 unsaturated fats. Shellfish, for example, clams, mussels, and mollusks, have solid advantages for your cerebrum and heart. Keep suppers fascinating by evaluating new plans.

- Stay in shape

Now that we have gone through the basics of the Mediterranean diet, we would love to journey with you on this quest. In this book, we provide recipes of meals that adhere to the Mediterranean diet for whatever time of the day.

Maybe perhaps the best quality of the Mediterranean eating routine is the way that it is exceptionally basic and direct. You don't should be a big name culinary expert to make the most delicious suppers; If you are wondering how you might scale through without repeating your meal plan every new week, then this book is for you.

All you have to do FLIP!

1.3 THE MEDITERRANEAN DIET PYRAMID

The Mediterranean diet is very simple to schematize. Using the image of a pyramid, one can be said that at the base of the diet is physical activity, which is the prerequisite for the body to stay healthy.

Nutrition is based on foods low in animal fats but rich in nutrients. At the base, there are cereals and vegetable oils. These foods must be consumed daily, on adequate portions, so that the body is equipped with enough energy to carry out its normal daily activities.

Going up the pyramid, we have vegetables and fruit. Plants, in particular, rich in vitamins, fiber, and minerals, poor in calories and fats, are fundamental for the well-being of the organism. Fruit also takes on the role of a healthy substitute for high-protein desserts (so to speak, a good fruit salad has no less flavor than a cake with cream, but it certainly has a clearly higher nutritional value).

We come now to protein intake. The Mediterranean diet guarantees high protein intake, obtained, however, not through red meat, but through fish, eggs, and poultry. White meats and eggs, so to speak, offer an excellent protein intake, but with a reduced intake of fats.

Going further up the pyramid, we find milk and its derivatives, certainly nutritious foods, but with a high intake of fats. These foods should, therefore, be consumed sparingly, as especially for those who have a sedentary lifestyle, they can represent enemies in the face of their fat intake.

Finally, we reach the top of the food pyramid of the Mediterranean diet. We find red meats and sweets. They are foods that must be limited, as they bring a very high amount of fat, and this can lead to numerous problems for the body.

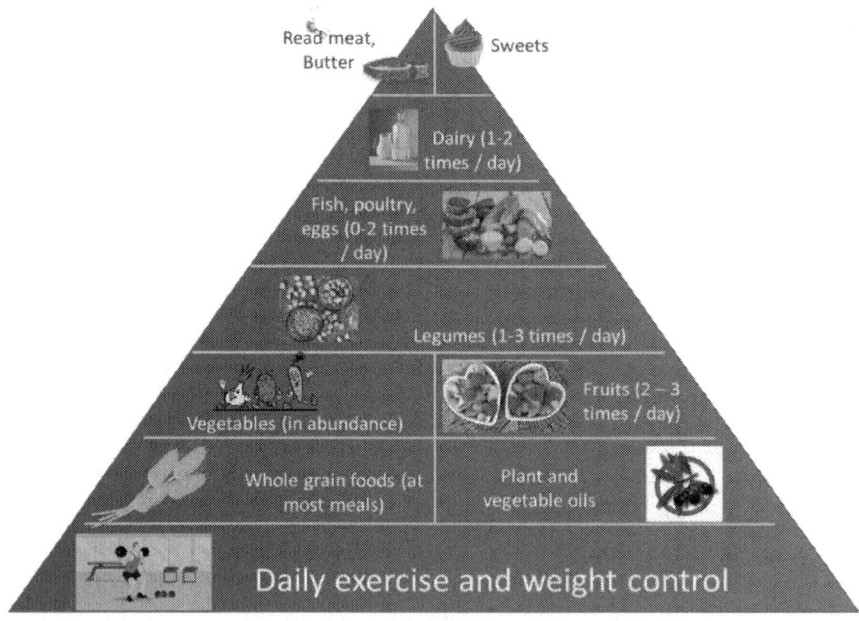

Looking at the pyramid, one can, therefore, understand what the weekly breakdown of types of food to be consumed must be. Premising the need for sport or, in any case, adequate physical activity, the consumption of food placed at the base of the pyramid must be preferred and be more careful in consuming food placed towards the top.

Here is a straightforward show you can utilize whenever you go food shopping:

•   Fruits: grapes, apples, berries, organic citrus products, avocado, bananas, papaya, pineapple, and so on.

•   Vegetables: broccoli, mushrooms, celery, carrots, kale, onions, leeks, eggplant, and so on.

•   Solidified vegetables: sound blended veggie alternatives, Vegetables: beans, lentils, peas, and so on.

•   Grains: every single entire grain including entire grain pasta and entire grain bread

•   Nuts: almonds, pecans, cashews, hazelnuts, pistachios, pine nuts, and so on.

•   Seeds: pumpkin, hemp, sesame, sunflower, and so on.

•   Fish: salmon, fish, herring, sardines, ocean bass, and so on.

•   Shellfish assortments and shrimp

•   "Free-range" chicken

- Baby Irish potatoes, sweet potatoes, and yams

- Cheddar

- Common Greek yogurt

- Olives

- Fed eggs

- Meat: goat, pork, and fed hamburger

- Additional virgin olive oil

1.4 THE MEAL PLAN

A necessary premise: before facing any change in your diet, you should consult with your doctor or nutritionist. This is because diets must be calibrated on the basis of personal physical characteristics and by virtue of the pathologies present.

For illustrative purposes, an exemplary scheme of the organization of meals within a week by adopting the Mediterranean diet is presented.

The structure of meals during the week follows the principle expressed by the food pyramid. As a consequence, it will be possible to observe a predominance of types of foods present at the base of the pyramid, while the foods present higher and higher in the pyramid will be consumed less frequently.

	MON	TUE	WED	THU	FRI	SAT	SUN
	BREAKFAST MEAL							
	SNACK							
LUNCH	PASTA	BREAD	RICE	PASTA	RICE	PASTA	PASTA
	RED MEAT	FISH	PORK / LAMB	POULTRY	FISH	RED MEAT	POULTRY
	VEGETABLES AND FRUITS							
	SNACK							
DINNER	SOUP	SOUP	SOUP	SOUP	SOUP	SOUP	
	EGGS	POULTRY	FISH	BREAD	POULTRY	CHEESE	PIZZA
	VEGETABLES AND FRUITS							

The Mediterranean diet includes three main meals (breakfast, lunch, and dinner) and two snacks. It is very important not to skip even one of the indicated meals. Dinner is generally very low in calories; on the contrary, breakfast, and lunch provide most of the nutrients and calories needed to face the day.

PART 2 – MEDITERRANEAN DIET RECIPES

2.1 LOAVES

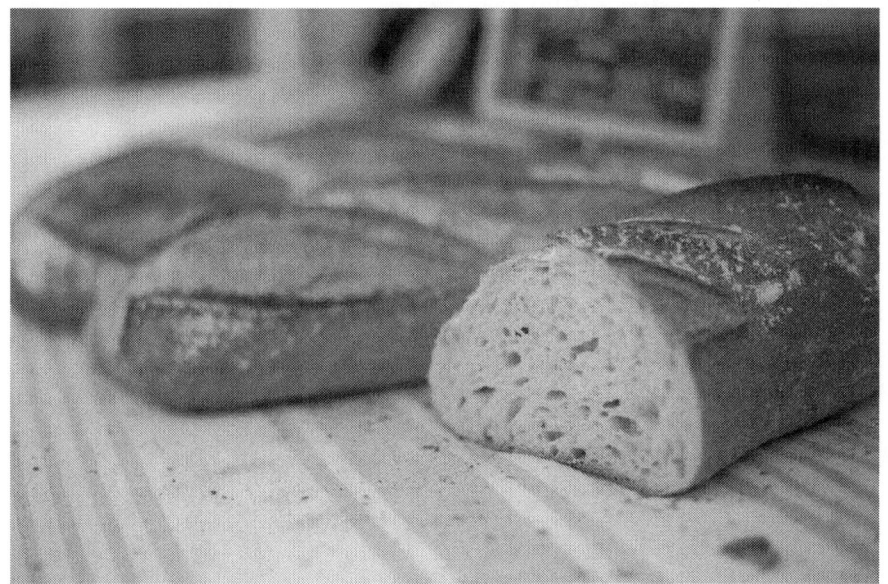

WHOLE WHEAT PITA BREAD

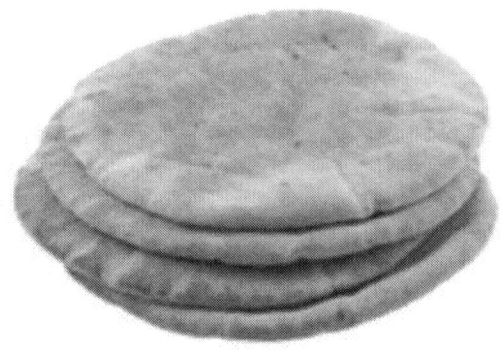

Makes 8 servings

FIXINGS

1 1/8 cups (265 ml) warm water
1 tablespoon (12 g) dynamic dry yeast
½ tablespoon (9 g) grungy ocean salt or on the other hand salt
2 cups (250 g) entire wheat flour
1½ cups (188 g) unbleached, generally useful flour
1 tablespoon (15 ml) extra-virgin olive oil

METHOD:

Empty the water into a huge bowl. Include the yeast and mix until broke down. Include the salt, and slowly consolidate the flours to frame a mixture. Turn the batter out onto a gently floured work surface and massage for 10 minutes, until smooth and versatile.

Or on the other hand place in the bowl of and electric blender fitted with a snare connection and work on medium speed for 2 minutes. Empty the oil into a bowl and spot batter inside the bowl, going to coat. Spread with oiled plastic and a kitchen towel and let ascend until multiplied in mass (1½ to 2 hours).

At the point when the batter has risen, punch down delicately. Gap the mixture into six equivalent parts and shape into balls. Spot on a daintily floured surface also, spread with a dry kitchen towel. Let rest for 15 minutes. Preheat the stove to 475°F (240°C). Spot a preparing stone or sheet in least segment of stove.

Reveal every mixture hover to shape a 6-inch (15 cm) circle. Spot three circles on the preheated preparing sheet and heat for around 12 minutes (until they are puffed up and start to turn shading). Cease from opening the stove during the initial 4 minutes of cooking.

Expel with a metal spatula or pizza strip and spot in a bread bushel or on a serving platter. Rehash with the rest of the batter hovers until all are prepared. In order to stay away from too much gluten, you can use alternative types of flour.

Supplant the flours in this formula with a mix of 1½ cups

(237 g) earthy colored rice flour, 1 cup (125 g) custard flour, 1 cup (136 g) sorghum flour, and additionally, 2 teaspoons of thickener- preferably xanthum gum

MEDITERRANEAN CORN BREAD

Makes 6-8 servings

Despite the fact that corn is local to the Americas, its ubiquity in the Mediterranean district is across the board to such an extent that you would think it started there. This Italian-propelled rendition is a refreshed understanding of conventional plans from the northern Italian districts.

Corn flour was called Turkish grains in Italian, and turned out to be very mainstream with the Jewish people group in Venice.

FIXINGS

2 teaspoons extra-virgin olive oil, separated
2½ cups (305 g) stone ground
100% entire grain, medium-crush cornmeal
½ tablespoon (9 g) grungy ocean salt or salt
2 teaspoons preparing powder
1 teaspoon sugar
2 cups (475 ml) bubbling water
¼ cup (14 g) hacked sun-dried tomatoes

4 ounces (115 g) new mozzarella cheddar, destroyed by hand into huge pieces

METHOD

Preheat the stove to 350°F (180°C). Oil a 8-inch (20 cm) round cake dish with 1 teaspoon olive oil. Consolidate the cornmeal, salt, staying 1 teaspoon olive oil, preparing powder, and sugar in a huge bowl.

Include the bubbling water and mix to blend until the entirety of the water is fused in the blend. Mix in the sun-dried tomatoes and mozzarella. Pour the cornmeal blend into the readied dish. Wet your hands and press down to smooth the top.

Prepare for 10 minutes and afterward spread the container with aluminum foil and prepare for 20 to 30 minutes, or until brilliant and firm on top. Permit to cool somewhat and serve warm, or permit to cool and envelop by cling wrap.

WHOLE WHEAT AND GRAPE FOCACCIA

Makes 8-10 servings.

This sort of bread is straightened out bread with fresh grapes squeezed into it .As indicated by realities, this formula began with the Etruscans and was heated in the cinders of an open hearth.

FIXINGS

1½ cups (425 ml) warm water
½ cup (120 ml) Vin Santo(Italian dessert wine)
1 bundle (¼ ounce, or 7 g) dynamic dry yeast
½ cup (118 ml) extra-virgin olive oil, partitioned, in addition to extra for lubing skillet
3 cups (375 g) entire wheat flour
1 cup (125 g) unbleached, universally handy flour
1 teaspoon foul ocean salt or salt
2 cups (300 g) seedless red grapes, cut down the middle the long way

METHOD

Pour the water and Vin Santo in the bowl of a standing blender. Sprinkle the yeast over the top, and blend utilizing the oar connection until joined. Let set for 5 minutes. Pour in ¼ cup (60 ml) of olive oil. Include the whole wheat flour and blend on low speed.

Gradually include the generally useful flour and salt, and blend until very much consolidated. Change to the mixture snare connection and ply the batter on medium speed for 5 minutes. Spread the bowl with oiled saran wrap and permit to rest at room temperature until multiplied in size, around 60 minutes. Oil a 13 x 17-inch (33 x 43 cm) rimmed heating sheet.

Turn the batter from the bowl onto the heating sheet. Stretch the batter out and press down until it covers the outside of the container in an even layer. Utilizing all the fingers of your hands, push down to make dimples in the surface of the focaccia.

Spread with oiled cling wrap and permit to rest for 30 minutes, or until the batter has multiplied in size once more. Preheat the stove to 425°F (220°C). Prior to preparing, brush the outside of the focaccia with the remaining ¼ cup (60 ml) of olive oil.

Disperse the grapes, chop side down ridiculous what's more, press them down somewhat. Heat for 30 to 35 minutes, or until the focaccia turns a decent brilliant earthy colored and is cooked through. Expel from the broiler and permit to cool somewhat. Cut and serve right away.

Extra, cooled pieces can be enveloped by cling wrap and

solidified for as long as multi month.

In case you are gluten intolerant, Dubstitute the flour in this formula with 1½ cups (188 g) custard flour, 1 1/3 cups (181 g) sorghum flour, 2/3 cup (129 g) potato starch, ½ cup (79 g) sweet rice flour, and 1 teaspoon thickener.

In the off chance that you might want to make this batter toward the beginning of the day to eat at night, spread the bowl with cling wrap and a spotless kitchen towel and spot in the fridge. In 12 hours, you will have indistinguishable outcomes from in the event that it sat at room temperature for 60 minutes.

BANANA-WALLNUT BREAD

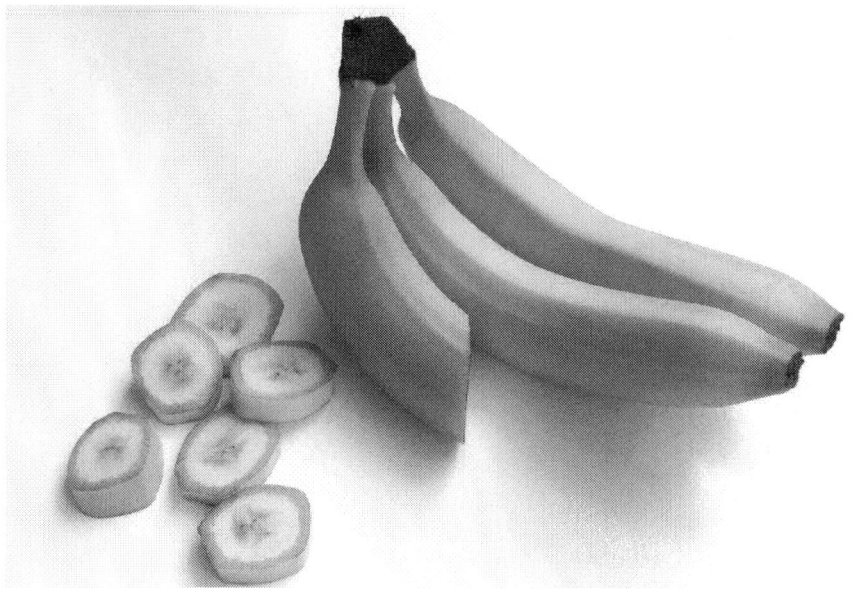

Makes 12 Cuts per Portion

FIXINGS

Canola oil cooking shower
1¾ cups generally useful flour
1½ teaspoons preparing pop
1½ teaspoons salt
3 huge eggs or ¾ cup fluid eggs
¾ cup low-calorie heating sugar
1 cup crushed exceptionally ready bananas (around 2 enormous bananas)
½ cup slashed pecans
½ cup canola oil

METHOD

Preheat stove to 350 degrees. Shower within a 9x5x3-inch heating portion skillet with cooking oil. Consolidate flour, heating pop, and salt in a bowl. Speed in eggs, sugar, bananas, pecans, and canola oil, and blend until all around mixed.

Scratch hitter into oiled portion container and heat for around an hour or until a toothpick embedded into the focal point of the portion tells the truth. Expel from broiler and spot skillet on a wire rack, permitting to cool for at any rate 15 minutes before attempting to discharge portion from the skillet.

SESAME BREAD

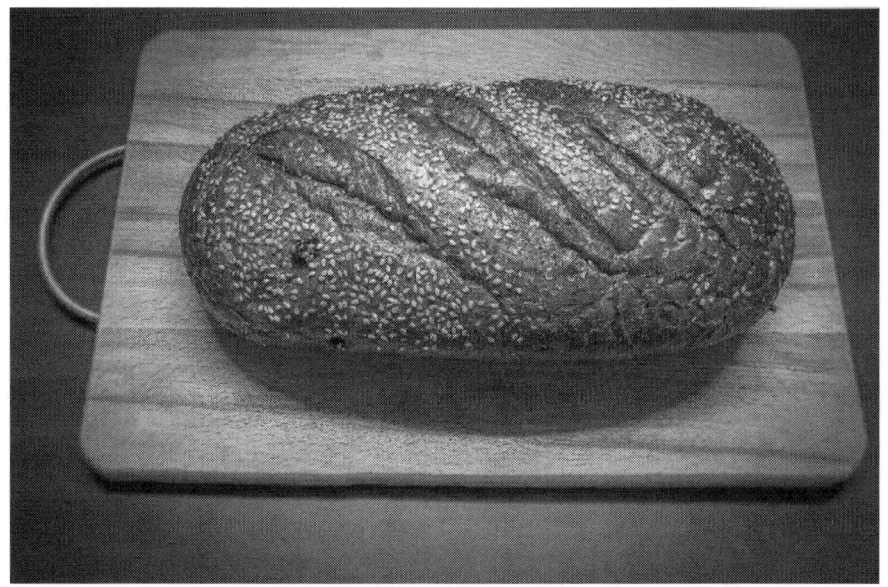

Makes 12 Cuts per Portion

Kersa is a round, level Moroccan bread that is marginally crunchy outwardly and chewy on the inside, extraordinary for dunking in soup or with stews.

FIXINGS

1 bundle of dynamic dry yeast ¼ cup
2 cups warm water
1 teaspoon low-calorie heating sugar
4 cups durum entire wheat semolina flour
2 teaspoons salt
⅓ cup cornmeal + extra for tidying

½ tablespoon extra-virgin olive oil
2 teaspoons sesame seeds

METHOD

Utilizing a little bowl, join yeast with ¼ cup water, include sugar, and let set until blend begins to bubble. In a substantial blender bowl with mixture snare blend flour, salt, and cornmeal. Indent focus of batter, pour in yeast blend and olive oil.

Work mixture, including remaining water varying until batter takes on a versatile quality. Oil 2 heating sheets and residue with cornmeal. Independent batter to shape 2 round balls and spot each ball on a different heating sheet. Press them into 8-inch circles.

Sprinkle 1 teaspoon of sesame seeds over each portion, delicately squeezing them into surface of batter. Spread mixture with a perfect fabric and put aside in a warm spot for around 1 hour until they twofold their size. Preheat broiler to 425 degrees.

Prick the highest point of portions with a fork and prepare for 10 minutes. Lower warmth to 375 degrees and heat portions until top is dried up and brilliant earthy colored, around 15–20 minutes.

NECTAR ENTIRE WHEAT BREAD

Makes 20–22 Cuts per Portion

FIXINGS

⅔ cup + 3 tablespoons water
2 tablespoons canola oil
1½ teaspoons without sodium salt substitute
1 tablespoon low-calorie earthy colored sugar mix
2 tablespoons common without fat dry milk
2 tablespoons unadulterated nectar
2¾ cups entire wheat flour
2¼ teaspoons dynamic dry yeast (at room temperature)

METHOD

If using a machine:

Expel preparing machine canister. To begin with, include water, at that point canola oil, salt substitute, sugar, milk, and nectar. Spread these fixings with flour lastly yeast. Try not to permit yeast to contact fluids.

Return canister to machine per machine guidelines, close cover, and adhere to setting directions for making entire wheat bread. At the point when machine is done, evacuate portion and permit to completely cool before cutting. Store any unused bread in cooler.

If Not:

Pre heat your oven to about 375 degrees follow the mixture of the fixings above and place into the oven. Leave there for about 30 minutes

WHOLE WHEAT NUTTY CRANBERRY BREAD

Makes 20–22 Cuts per Portion

FIXINGS

¾ cup + 7 tablespoons water
2 tablespoons canola oil
1½ teaspoons sans sodium salt substitute
2 tablespoons low-calorie earthy colored sugar mix
2 tablespoons normal without fat dry milk
2¾ cups entire wheat flour
½ cup slashed dried cranberries
¼ cup cut crude almonds
2¼ teaspoons dynamic dry yeast (at room temperature)

METHOD

Evacuate preparing machine canister. Initially, include water, at that point canola oil, salt substitute, sugar, and milk. Spread fluid fixings with flour, cranberries, nuts, lastly yeast. Try not to permit yeast to contact fluids.

Return canister to machine per machine directions, close top, and adhere to setting guidelines for making entire wheat bread. At the point when machine is done, expel portion what's more, permit to completely cool before cutting. Store any unused bread in cooler.

NATURAL WHOLE WHEAT BREAD

Makes 20–22 Cuts per Portion

FIXINGS.

1¼ cups of water
2 tablespoons canola oil
1½ teaspoons sans sodium salt substitute
2 tablespoons low-calorie earthy colored sugar mix
2 tablespoons regular sans fat dry milk 2¾ cups entire wheat flour
⅓ cup gently salted pumpkin seeds
5 dried apricots, finely cleaved
¼ cup white raisins
¼ cup cut crude almonds
2¼ teaspoons dynamic dry yeast (at room temperature)

METHOD

Evacuate heating machine canister. To start with, include water, at that point canola oil, salt substitute, sugar, and milk. Spread these fixings with flour, seeds, apricots, raisins, almonds, lastly yeast.

Try not to permit yeast to contact fluids. Return canister to machine per machine directions, close top, and follow setting directions for making entire wheat bread. At the point when machine is completed, evacuate portion and permit to altogether cool before cutting. Store any unused bread in cooler.

WHOLE WHEAT BREAD (NUTTY POMEGRANTE)

Makes 20–22 Cuts per Portion

FIXINGS

1¼ cups of water
2 tablespoons canola oil

1½ teaspoons without sodium salt substitute
2 tablespoons low-calorie earthy colored sugar mix

2 tablespoons characteristic dry milk

2¾ cups entire wheat flour

Seeds from 1 pomegranate natural product

⅓ cup daintily salted pumpkin seeds

¼ cup cut crude almonds

1½ teaspoons dried orange strip

2¼ teaspoons dynamic dry yeast (at room temperature)

METHOD

Expel preparing machine canister. To begin with, include water, at that point canola oil, salt substitute, sugar, and milk. Spread these fixings with flour, pomegranate and pumpkin seeds, almonds, orange strip, and at last yeast. Try not to permit yeast to contact fluids.

Return canister to machine per machine directions, close cover, and adhere to setting guidelines for making entire wheat bread. At the point when machine is done, expel portion what's more, permit to altogether cool before cutting. Store any unused bread in cooler.

WHOLE WHEAT BREAD (NUTTY)

Makes 20–22 Cuts per Portion

FIXINGS

1¼ cups of water
2 tablespoons canola oil
1½ teaspoons sans sodium salt substitute
2 tablespoons low-calorie earthy colored sugar mix
2 tablespoons regular sans fat dry milk
2¾ cups entire wheat flour
¼ cup finely cleaved crude pecans
1½ teaspoons dried orange strip
⅓ cup gently salted pumpkin seeds
2¼ teaspoons dynamic dry yeast (at room temperature)

METHOD

Evacuate heating machine canister. To begin with, include water, at that point canola oil, salt substitute, sugar, and milk. Spread these fixings with flour, nuts, orange strip, seeds, lastly yeast. Try not to permit yeast to contact fluids.

Return canister to machine per machine guidelines, close top, and adhere to setting guidelines for making entire wheat bread. When machine is done, evacuate portion and permit to completely cool previously cutting. Store any unused bread in cooler.

SUNDRIED TOMATO BASIL WHITE WHEAT BREAD

Makes 20–22 Cuts per Portion

1½ cups water (room temperature)
2 tablespoons olive oil
2 teaspoons without sodium salt substitute
3 tablespoons low-calorie earthy colored sugar mix
3 tablespoons normal sans fat dry milk
3 tablespoons new sundried tomato pesto
8 huge pitted dark olives, slashed
10 sundried tomatoes, hacked
2 cups white wheat flour
2 cups bread flour
2 teaspoons dynamic dry yeast

METHOD

Expel preparing machine canister. To begin with, include water, at that point canola oil, salt substitute, sugar, milk, pesto, olives, and sundried tomatoes. Spread these fixings with the two flours lastly yeast. Try not to permit yeast to contact fluids.

Return canister to machine per machine directions, close top, and adhere to setting guidelines for making white wheat bread. At the point when machine is done, expel portion and permit to completely cool before cutting. Store any unused bread in cooler.

WHOLE WHEAT MORROCCAN BREAD

Makes 3 Portions

This simple bread, frequently made with grain, has a delicate, sodden morsel. It is a Moroccan formula, and it's an extraordinary bread for any feast. It is best eaten the day it is made, or solidified at that point defrosted and warmed the day it is served.

FIXINGS

2½ cups (570 ml) warm water
1 tablespoon (12 g) dynamic, dry yeast
2 teaspoons sugar
1 teaspoon legitimate salt
6 to 8 cups (750 g to 1kg) whole wheat or on the other hand grain flour, in addition to extra for working
4 teaspoons (20 ml) extra-virgin olive oil, separated
3 teaspoons (8 g) sesame seeds

METHOD

Empty the warm water into the bowl of a standing electric blender with a paddle connection. Sprinkle the yeast and sugar over the water, and blend until broke up. Include the salt and steadily blend in 6 cups (750 g) of flour, signifying 2 additional cups, one cup (125 g) at once, until batter pulls away from the side of the bowl.

Change to a snare connection and work for 5 minutes on medium speed, or until smooth. Fold the batter into a 12-inch (30 cm) log, at that point separate into three equivalent pieces. Shape each piece into a 4-inch (10 cm) arch molded portion. Spot portions on a heating sheet lubed with 1 teaspoon oil. Spread with a kitchen towel and spot in a without draft region to ascend for 60 minutes, or until multiplied. Preheat the stove to 350°F (180°C).

Reveal the portions and brush each with 1 teaspoon olive oil and 1 teaspoon sesame seeds. Prepare for 20 to 30 minutes, or until delicately brilliant. Let cool somewhat, and serve warm. Freeze by enclosing it by cling wrap and afterward aluminum foil.

Defrost at room temperature and warm in a preheated 350°F (180°C) stove before serving.

2.2 BREAKFAST MEALS

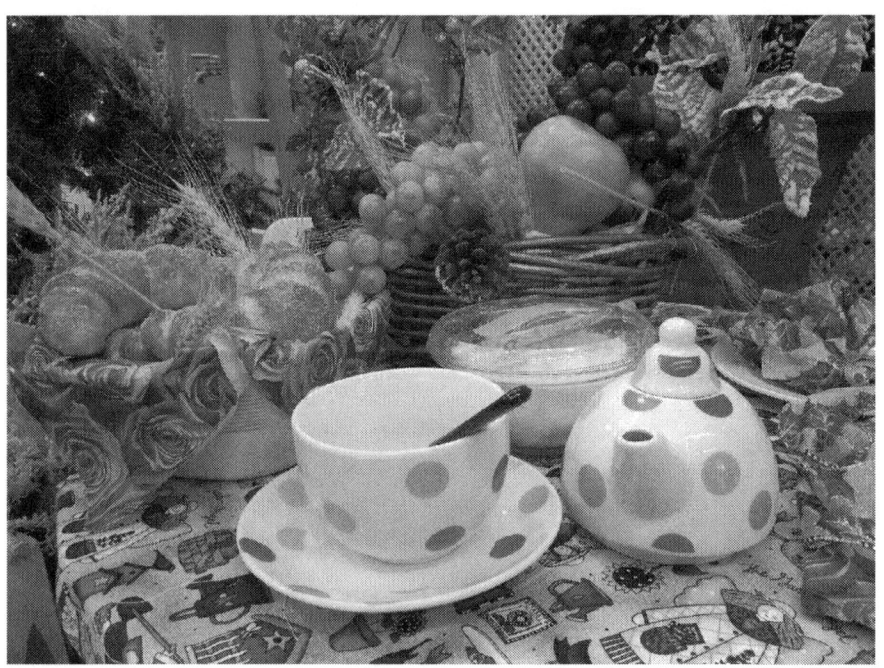

BREAKFAST WRAP

Makes 2 servings

FIXINGS

½ cup new picked spinach
4 egg whites
2 Bella sun-dried tomatoes
2 blended grain flax wraps

½ cup feta cheddar disintegrates

METHOD

Cook spinach, egg whites and tomatoes in a griddle for around 4 minutes or then again until gently carmelized .Flip it over and cook the opposite side for 4 minutes or until nearly done.

Microwave the wraps for around 15 seconds; expel from the microwave, fill each wrap with the egg blend, sprinkle with feta cheddar disintegrates and move up. Cut each wrap into two sections and serve.

BREAKFAST CASSEROLE

Makes 6 servings

FIXINGS

2 tbsp. additional virgin olive oil, isolated
½ a medium-sized onion, diced
2 medium-sized yellow potatoes. diced
1 lb. zucchini, cut
3 portabella mushroom tops, diced
150g torn new spinach

200g ricotta
200g light ricotta cheddar
2 cups of egg whites
12 grape tomatoes, sliced into ⅓ pieces
3 stripped and simmered new peppers, cut
2 sourdough rolls
4 tbsp. Pecorino Romano cheddar, ground
100g skim-milk mozzarella cheddar, ground

METHOD

Preheat the broiler to 400°F. Combine olive oil, onion and potato and meal for in any event 15 minutes; expel from broiler and keep on the preparing plate. In a bowl, join together ½ tablespoon olive oil and zucchini; hurl to coat well and move to a heating plate.

Return all the vegetables to broiler and dish for around 40 minutes or until brilliant in shading. Meanwhile, place ½ tablespoon olive oil in a dish and sauté mushrooms for around 4 minutes.

Expel the cooked mushrooms from container and put in a safe spot. Add the staying olive oil to container and sauté hacked spinach until delicate. In a blending bowl, join together the two kinds of ricotta and egg whites; set aside.

Join together all the vegetables, including grape tomatoes and peppers, with sourdough overflows with a 9 x 13 heating dish; top with the ricotta blend also, sprinkle with pecorino and mozzarella cheddar.

Prepare for in any event 40 minutes or until done. Expel from the broiler, cool somewhat. Cut into six cuts and make the most of your morning meal

COUSCOUS

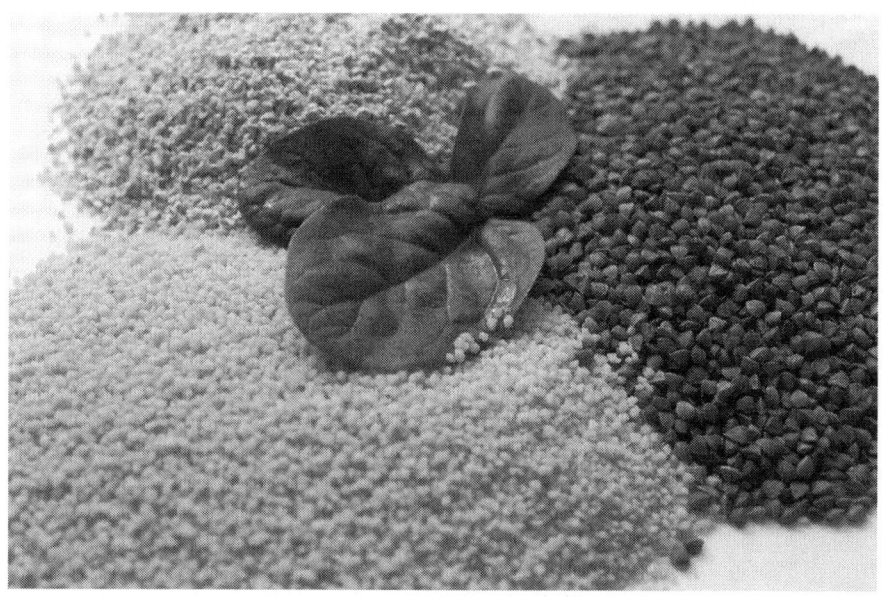

Makes 4 servings.

FIXINGS

1 (2-inch) cinnamon stick
3 cups 1% low-fat milk
1 cup entire wheat couscous (uncooked)
6 tsp. dim earthy colored sugar, partitioned
¼ cup dried currants
½ cup hacked apricots (dried)
¼ tsp. ocean salt
4 tsp. dissolved spread, isolated

METHOD

In a pot set over medium high warmth, consolidate cinnamon stick and milk; heat for around 3 minutes (don't bubble). Expel the skillet from warmth and mix in couscous, 4 teaspoons of sugar, currants, apricots, and ocean salt.

Allow the blend to stand, secured, for in any event 15 minutes. Dispose of the cinnamon stick and separation the couscous among four dishes; top each presenting with ½ teaspoon of sugar and 1 teaspoon of dissolved margarine. Serve right away

MEDITERRANEAN PANCAKES

Makes 16 pieces.

FIXINGS.

1 cup antiquated oats
½ cup generally useful flour
2 tbsp. flax seeds
1 tsp. preparing pop
¼ tsp. ocean salt
2 tbsp. additional virgin olive oil
2 huge eggs
2 cups nonfat plain Greek yogurt
2 tbsp. crude nectar
New natural product, syrup, or different fixings

METHODS

In a blender, consolidate oats, flour, flax seeds, preparing pop, and ocean salt; mix for around 30 seconds. Include additional virgin olive oil, eggs, yogurt, and nectar and keep beating until exceptionally smooth.

Let the blend represent in any event 20 minutes or until thick. Set a huge nonstick skillet over medium warmth and brush with additional virgin olive oil. In bunches, spoon the player by quarter-cupfuls into the skillet.

Cook the flapjacks for around 2 minutes or until bubbles structure and brilliant earthy colored. Turn them over and cook different sides for 2 minutes more or until brilliant earthy colored. Serve!

Note: Gluten-free alternatives are listed above, in case it is needed.

MEDITERRANEAN FRITTATA

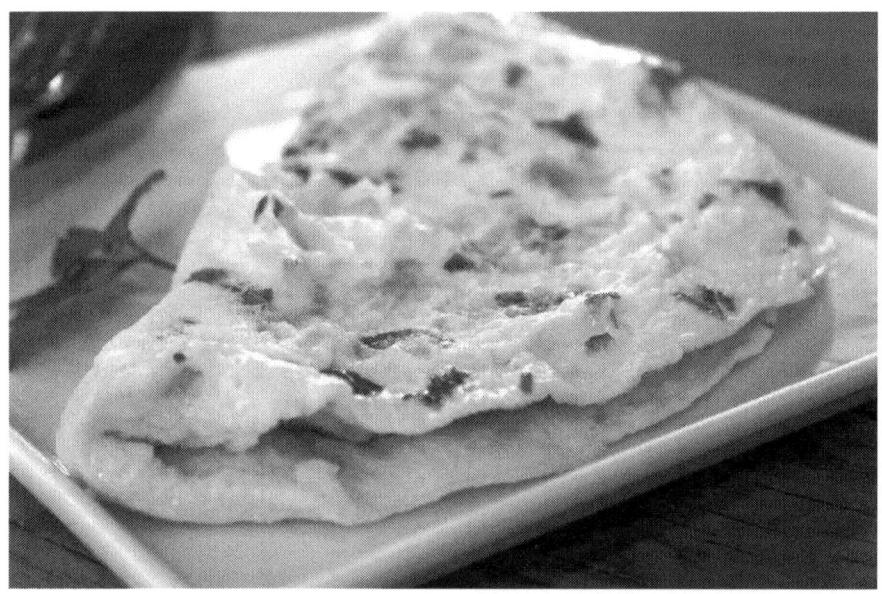

Makes 4 servings

FIXINGS

3 tbsp. additional virgin olive oil, separated
1 cup cleaved onion
2 cloves garlic, minced
8 eggs, beaten
¼ cup creamer, milk or light cream
½ cup cut Kalamata olives
½ cup cooked red sweet peppers, hacked
½ cup disintegrated feta cheddar
⅛ tsp. dark pepper
¼ cup new basil
2 tbsp. Parmesan cheddar, finely destroyed
½ cup coarsely squashed onion-and-garlic bread garnishes
Fresh basil leaves, to embellish

METHOD

Preheat your oven. Warmth 2 tablespoons of additional virgin olive oil in an oven verification skillet set over medium warmth; sauté onion and garlic for a couple of moments or until delicate. Meanwhile, beat eggs and creamer in a bowl until very much joined.

Mix in olives, cooked sweet pepper, feta cheddar, dark pepper and basil. Pour the egg blend over the sautéed onion blend and cook until nearly set.

With a spatula, lift the egg blend to permit the uncooked part to stream underneath.

Keep cooking for 2 minutes more or until the set. Consolidate the staying additional virgin olive oil, Parmesan cheddar, and squashed bread garnishes in a bowl; sprinkle the blend over the frittata and sear for about 5 minutes or until the pieces are brilliant and the top is set.

To serve, cut the frittata into wedges and trimming with new basil.

BANANA OATMEAL (NUTTY)

Makes four servings

FIXINGS

¼ cup speedy cooking oats
3 tbsp. crude nectar
½ cup skim milk
2 tbsp. hacked pecans
1 tsp. flax seeds
1 banana, stripped

METHOD

In a microwave-safe bowl, consolidate oats, nectar, milk,

pecans, and flaxseeds; microwave on high for around 2 minutes. In a little bowl, crush the banana with a fork to a fine consistency; mix into the oats and serve hot.

MEDITERRANEAN VEGGIE OMELET

Makes 4 servings

FIXINGS

1 tbsp. additional virgin olive oil
2 cups daintily cut new fennel bulb
¼ cup hacked artichoke hearts, absorbed water, depleted
¼ cup pitted green olives, salt water relieved, hacked
1 diced Roma tomato
6 eggs
¼ tsp. ocean salt
½ tsp. newly ground dark pepper
½ cup goat cheddar, disintegrated
2 tbsp. newly hacked new parsley, dill, or basil

METHOD

Preheat your stove to 325°F. Warmth additional virgin olive oil in an ovenproof skillet over medium warmth. Sauté fennel for around 5 minutes or until delicate. Include artichoke hearts, olives, and tomatoes and cook for 3minutes metal or until mollified.

In a bowl, beat the eggs; season with ocean salt and pepper. Include the egg blend over the vegetables and mix for around 2 minutes. Sprinkle cheddar over the omelet and prepare in the stove for around 5 minutes or until set and cooked through.

Top with parsley, dill, or basil. Move the omelet onto a cutting board, painstakingly cut into four wedges, also, serve right away.

AVOCADO TOAST

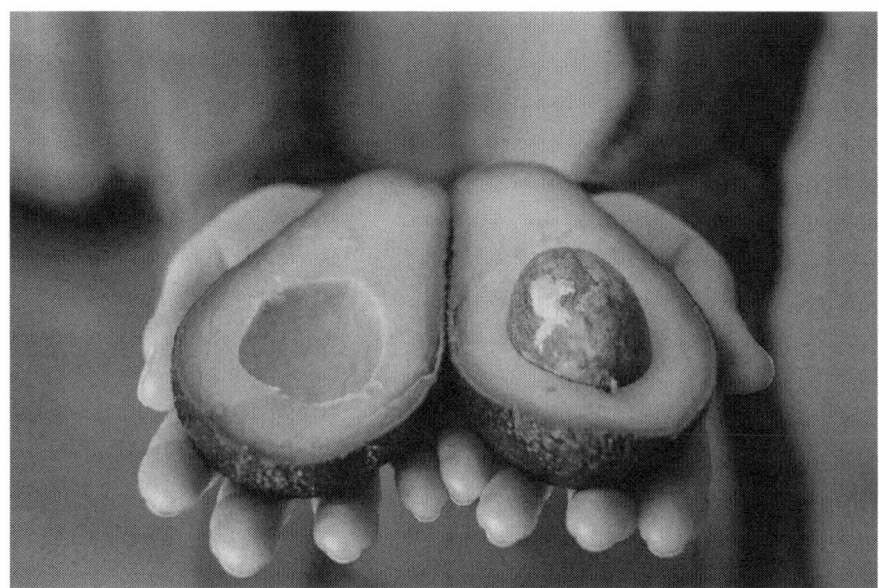

Makes 4 Servings

FIXINGS

2 ready avocados, stripped
Crush of new lemon juice, to taste
2 tbsp. newly slashed mint, in addition to extra to embellish
Ocean salt and dark pepper, to taste
4 enormous cuts rye bread
80 grams delicate feta, disintegrated

METHOD

In a medium bowl, pound the avocado generally with a fork; include lemon juice what's more, mint and keep squashing until simply joined. Season with dark pepper and ocean salt to taste. Flame broil or toast bread until brilliant. Spread about ¼ of the avocado blend onto each cut of the toasted bread what's more, top with feta. Embellishment with additional mint and serve right away.

LEMON SCONES

Makes 12 servings

FIXINGS

2 cups in addition to ¼ cup flour
½ tsp. preparing pop
2 tbsp. sugar
½ tsp. ocean salt
¾ cup decreased fat buttermilk
Get-up-and-go of 1 lemon
1 to 2 tsp. newly pressed lemon juice
1 cup powdered sugar

METHOD

Preheat your oven to 400°F. In a food processor, consolidate 2 cups of flour, heating pop, sugar and salt until all around mixed. Include buttermilk and lemon get-up-and-go and keep blending to join well.

Sprinkle the rest of the flour onto a clear surface and turn out the batter; tenderly ply the mixture in any event multiple times and shape it into a ball. Utilizing a moving pin, level the batter into half-inch thick circle. Cut the batter into four equivalent wedges and the cut each into three littler wedges.

Orchestrate the scones on a preparing sheet and heat in preheated stove for about 15 minutes or until brilliant earthy colored. Combine lemon juice and the powdered sugar in a little bowl to make a flimsy icing. Expel the scones from the broiler and sprinkle with lemon icing while still hot. Serve immediately.

SCRAMBLED EGG (GARLIC ENHANCED)

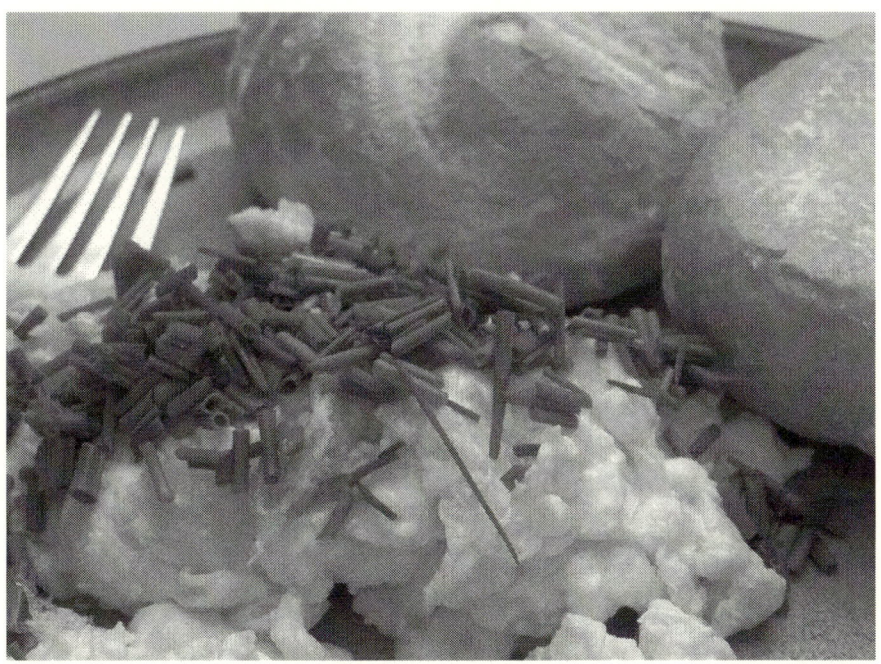

Makes 2 servings

FIXINGS

½ tsp. additional virgin olive oil
½ cup ground meat
½ tsp. garlic powder
3 eggs
Salt
Pepper

METHOD

Set a medium-sized dish over medium warmth. Include additional virgin olive oil and warmth until hot yet not smoking. Mix in ground meat and cook for around 10 minutes or until nearly done.

Mix in garlic and sauté for around 2 minutes. In an enormous bowl, beat the eggs until practically foamy; season with salt and pepper. Add the egg blend to the container with the cooked hamburger and scramble until prepared.

Present with toasted bread and olives, for a solid, fulfilling breakfast!

EGG AND SUASAGE CASSEROLE

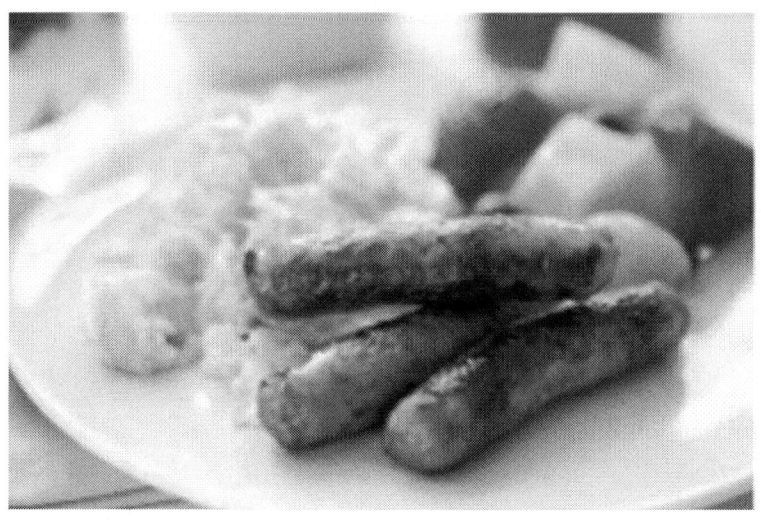

Makes 12 Servings

FIXINGS

For Crust:

3 tbsp. olive oil, separated
2 lb. stripped and destroyed reddish brown potatoes
¾ tsp. ground pepper
¾ tsp. salt

For Dish:

12 oz. hacked turkey frankfurter
4 daintily cut green onions
¼ cup diced chime pepper

⅓ cup skim milk
6 huge eggs
4 egg whites
¾ cup destroyed cheddar
16 oz. low-fat curds

METHOD

For Crust:

Preheat the stove to 425°F. Gently oil a 9×13-inch preparing dish with 1 tbsp. olive oil and put in a safe spot. Press abundance dampness out of the potato with a kitchen towel or paper towel.

Hurl together the potatoes, the staying olive oil, salt and pepper in a medium bowl until potatoes are all around covered. Move the blend to the lubed heating dish; equally press the blend up the sides and on the base of the dish and prepare for around 20 minutes or until brilliant earthy colored on the edges.

The Dish:

Lessen the stove warmth to 375°F. In an enormous skillet, cook turkey hotdog over medium-high warmth for around 2 minutes or until it's nearly cooked through. Include green onions and red ringer pepper and keep cooking for 2 more minutes or until ringer pepper is delicate.

Whisk together skim milk, eggs, egg whites, and the cheeses. Mix in turkey frankfurter blend; pour over the potato hull and prepare for around 50 minutes. Marginally cool and cut into 12 pieces, and serve.

YOGURT PANCAKES

Makes 5 Servings

FIXINGS

Whole wheat pancake blend
1 cup yogurt
1 tbsp. preparing powder
1 tbsp. preparing pop
1 cup skimmed milk
3 entire eggs
½ tsp. additional virgin olive oil

METHODS

Join together entire wheat flapjack blend, yogurt, heating powder, heating pop, skimmed milk and eggs in huge bowl. Mix until very much mixed. Warmth a skillet oiled daintily with olive oil.

Pour ¼ cup player onto the warmed container and cook for around 2 minutes or until the outside of the hotcake has a few air pockets. Flip and keep cooking until the underside is carmelized.

Serve the hotcakes warm with some sans fat milk or two tablespoons light maple syrup.

BREAKFAST SAUTEED FOOD

Makes 4 Servings

FIXINGS

1 tbsp. additional virgin olive oil
2 green peppers, cut
2 little onions, finely cleaved
4 tomatoes, cleaved
½ tsp. ocean salt
1 egg

METHODS

Warmth olive oil in a medium-sized container over medium-high warmth. Include green pepper and sauté for around 2 minutes. Lower warmth to medium and keep cooking, secured, for 3 additional minutes.

Mix in onion and cook for around 2 minutes or until earthy colored. Mix in tomatoes and salt; spread and stew to get a delicate delicious blend. In a bowl, beat the egg; sprinkle over the tomato blend and cook for about 1 moment. (Try not to mix).

Present with cleaved cucumbers, feta cheddar and dark olives for an extraordinary breakfast!

GREEK BREAKFAST PITAS

Makes 4 servings

FIXINGS

¼ cup cleaved onion
¼ cup sweet red/dark pepper, cleaved
1 cup enormous egg
⅛ tsp. ocean salt
⅛ tsp. dark pepper
1 ½ tsp. new basil, ground
½ cup infant spinach, newly torn
1 red tomato, cut

2 pita bread, entirety
2 tbsp. feta cheddar, disintegrated

METHODS

Coat a sizeable nonstick skillet with cooking shower and set over medium heat. Include onions and red peppers and sauté for at any rate 3 minutes. In a little bowl, beat together egg, pepper and salt and add the blend to the skillet.

Cook, blending persistently, until prepared. Spoon basil, spinach, and tomatoes onto the pitas and top with the egg blend. Sprinkle with feta and serve.

BREAKFAST SCRAMBLE

Makes 2 servings

FIXINGS

1 tsp. additional virgin olive
4 medium green onions, hacked
1 tsp. dried basil leaves or 1 tbsp. new basil leaves, hacked
1 medium tomato, hacked
4 eggs

fresh ground pepper

METHODS

In a medium nonstick skillet, heat olive oil over medium warmth; sauté green onions, mixing periodically, for around 2 minutes. Mix in basil and tomato and let cook, mixing periodically, for around 1 minute or until the tomato is cooked through.

In a little bowl, altogether beat the eggs with a wire whisk or a fork and pour over the tomato blend; cook for around 2 minutes. Tenderly lift the cooked parts with spatula to permit the uncooked parts to stream to the base.

Keep cooking for around 3 minutes or until the eggs are cooked through. Season with pepper and serve.

GREEK PARFAIT

Makes 6 servings

FIXINGS

1 tsp. vanilla concentrate
3 cups low-fat Greek yogurt

¼ cup toasted unsalted pistachios, shelled
4 tsp. crude nectar
28 Clementine portions

METHODS

In a blending bowl, consolidate the vanilla concentrate with the Greek yogurt. Spoon ¼ cup of the blend into 4 little parfait glasses. Top every one of the 4 glasses with ½ tablespoon nuts, ½ teaspoon nectar and 5 Clementine areas.

Add the rest of the yogurt blend to the parfait glasses and top with ½ tablespoon nuts, Clementine fragments and ½ teaspoon nectar. Serve right away

QUICHE ENVELOPED BY PROSCIUTTO

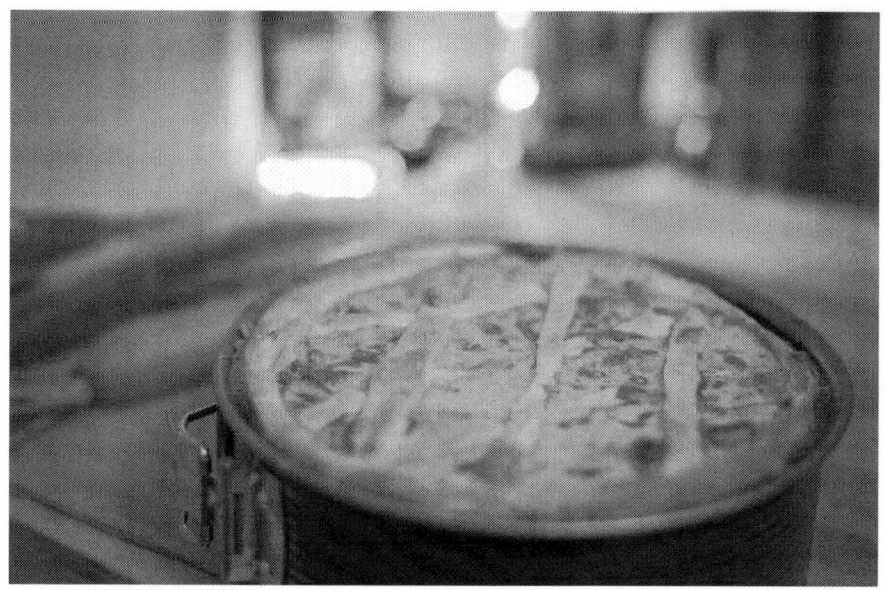

Makes 8 servings

FIXINGS

4 cuts prosciutto, split
2 egg whites
1 egg
½ tsp. rosemary, new and hacked and somewhat more for decorating
3 tbsp. low fat Greek yogurt
1 tbsp. hacked dark olives
A touch of dark pepper, newly ground
A touch of salt

METHODS

Preheat your stove to 400°F and cover your biscuit heating plate with cooking shower.
Spot every prosciutto piece into eight cups of the plate. In a medium bowl, whisk the egg whites and the egg until smooth.

Pour in the yogurt, rosemary, olives, pepper, and salt and proceed whisking. Partition the blend similarly among the prosciutto cups and prepare revealed until cooked through (around 15 minutes).

GREEN OMELET

Makes 4 servings

FIXINGS

8 eggs
yellow onion, finely slashed
1 clove garlic, minced
1 medium bundle of collard greens
3 tbsp. parsley, slashed
1 tsp. allspice
5 tbsp. additional virgin olive oil
½ cup Parmigiano-Reggiano cheddar, ground
1 squeeze ocean salt, discretionary

METHOD

Beat the eggs in a major bowl and include the onion, garlic, collard greens, parsley, and allspice. Keep beating until all the fixings blend well. Put a nonstick skillet on medium warmth and pour in the olive oil until hot Include the substance of the bowl and let cook for around 5 minutes or until it turns brilliant earthy colored.

Utilize a spatula to flip the omelet and cook the opposite side for 5 minutes or until it turns brilliant earthy colored. Serve on a plate, cut into wanted parts, at that point sprinkle the ground cheddar what's more. Enjoy!

QUINOA

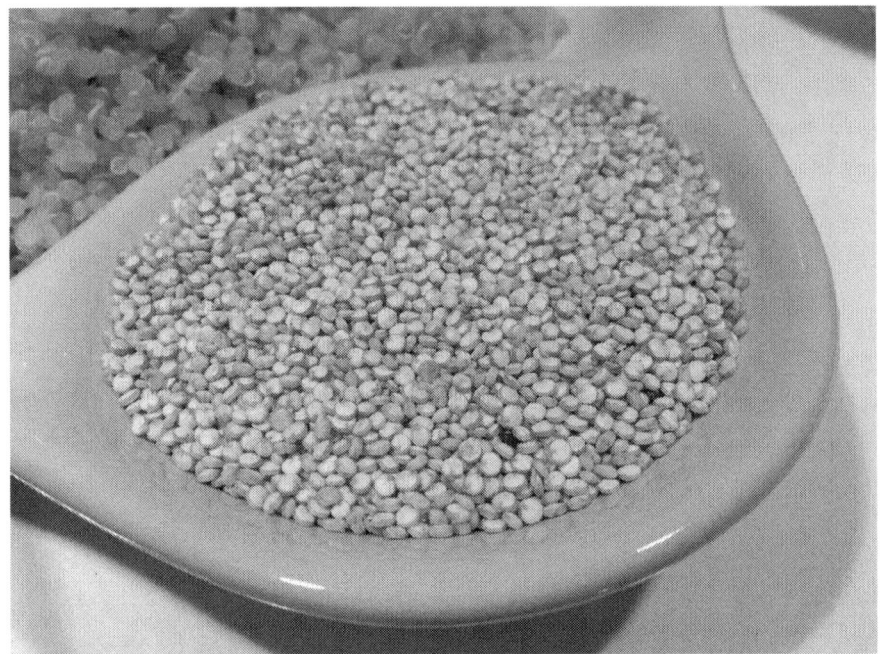

Makes 4 servings

FIXINGS

1 cup almonds
1 tsp. ground cinnamon
1 cup quinoa
2 cups milk
1 squeeze ocean salt
2 tbsp. nectar
5 dried apricots, finely hacked
2 dried, pitted dates, finely hacked
1 tsp. vanilla concentrate

METHOD

Start by toasting the almonds on a skillet for five minutes or until brilliant earthy colored for a decent nutty flavor. Spot a pot over medium warmth and include the quinoa and cinnamon; heat until warmed through.

Follow by including the milk and ocean salt while mixing from the beginning. When the blend reaches boiling point, lessen the warmth, spread the pot and let it stew for 15 minutes.

Include the nectar, apricots, dates, vanilla concentrate and a large portion of the almonds into the pan. Serve in bowls and top with the rest of the almonds

PROTEIN BARS

Makes 6 Servings

FIXINGS

¼ cup walnuts, slashed
2 tbsp. pistachios, slashed
¼ cup flaxseeds, ground
1 ¼ cup spelt drops

½ cup dried fruits
1 squeeze ocean salt
½ cup nectar
2 tbsp. additional virgin olive oil
¼ cup nutty spread, regular
½ tsp. vanilla concentrate

METHOD

Start by preheating your broiler to 325°F, at that point brush your heating plate with oil.
Line the heating plate with material paper all round and brush it with oil. Join the walnuts, pistachios, flaxseeds, spelt, fruits, and salt in a blending bowl and put in a safe spot.

Spot a pan over medium warmth and pour in the nectar, oil, nut margarine, and vanilla concentrate and cook, blending, until the blend softens. Add this blend to the bowl of dry fixings and blend well. Empty the blend into the readied heating plate and smooth the top.

Heat until it turns brilliant earthy colored and the sides pull out from the edges of the dish. Move the prepared bar from the plate and cut it into littler sizes on a cutting board. Subsequent to cooling, store in a water/air proof holder fixed with material paper.

The bars can last as long as a week.

2.3 MEDITERREANEAN DIET SALADS

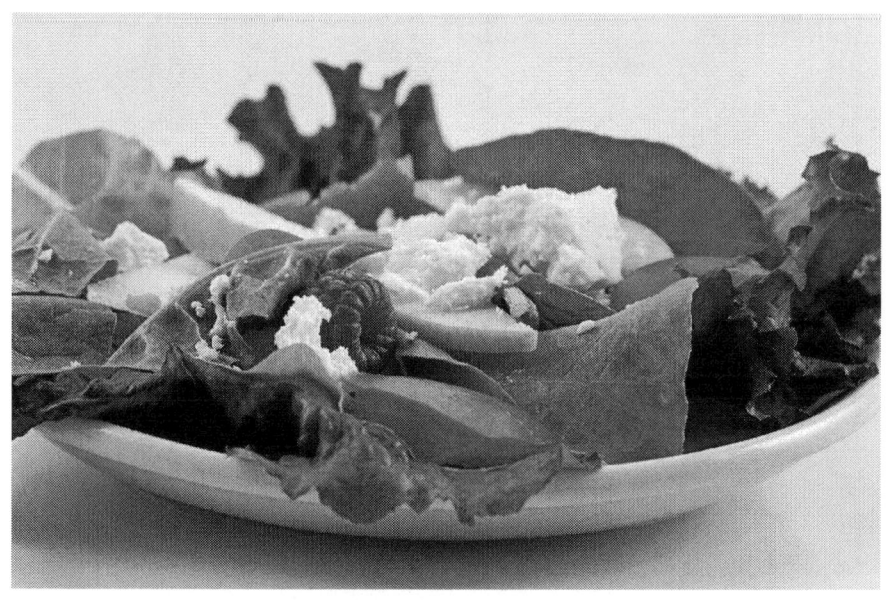

GREEK OLIVE AND FETA CHEDDAR PASTA

Makes 4 Servings

FIXINGS

4½ ounces ziti pasta
3 ounces disintegrated feta cheddar
10 little Greek olives, pitted and coarsely hacked ¼ cup new, coarsely hacked basil leaves
2 cloves new garlic, finely minced
1 tablespoon extra-virgin olive oil + more to shower ¼ teaspoon finely hacked hot pepper

½ red chime pepper, diced
½ yellow chime pepper, diced
2 plum tomatoes, seeded and diced

METHOD

Heat water to the point of boiling. Add pasta, and cook pasta until still somewhat firm. Expel from heat, channel pasta, and come back to pot, showering with insufficient measure of olive oil to shield pasta from staying together. Put in a safe spot.

In an enormous serving bowl join feta cheddar, olives, basil, garlic, olive oil, and hot pepper, at that point put in a safe spot for 30 minutes. Include cooked pasta, red and yellow chime peppers, and tomatoes; hurl fixings well.

Cover and refrigerate for in any event 60 minutes, until very much chilled. Hurl again before serving. This plate of mixed greens works out in a good way as a side dish to flame broiled sheep or fish.

GOAT CHEDDAR STUFFED TOMATOES

Makes 2 Servings

6–8 leaves arugula
2 medium ready tomatoes
3 ounces disintegrated feta cheddar
Salt and newly ground pepper to taste
Balsamic vinegar to sprinkle
Extra-virgin olive oil to sprinkle
1 red onion, meagerly cut for decorate
New cleaved parsley for decorate

METHOD

Spot 3–4 leaves arugula in the focal point of every serving of mixed greens plate. Cut tops (about ¼ inch) off the tomatoes. With a paring blade, center out the focal point of the tomatoes, about ½ inch down.

Fill tomatoes with disintegrated feta cheddar, include salt and pepper to taste, and shower with balsamic vinegar and olive oil. Enhancement with red onion cuts and hacked parsley. Serve at room temperature.

SYRIAN CUCUMBER AND YOGURT

Makes 4 Servings

FIXINGS

1½ teaspoons squashed new garlic
⅛ teaspoon minced new dill Salt to taste
1 quart plain low-fat yogurt
2 English cucumbers, stripped and diced
2 tablespoons dried mint

METHOD

In a bowl consolidate garlic, dill, and salt. Include yogurt and blend well. Mix in cucumbers and mint. Cover and refrigerate until very much chilled before serving.

TABBOULEH

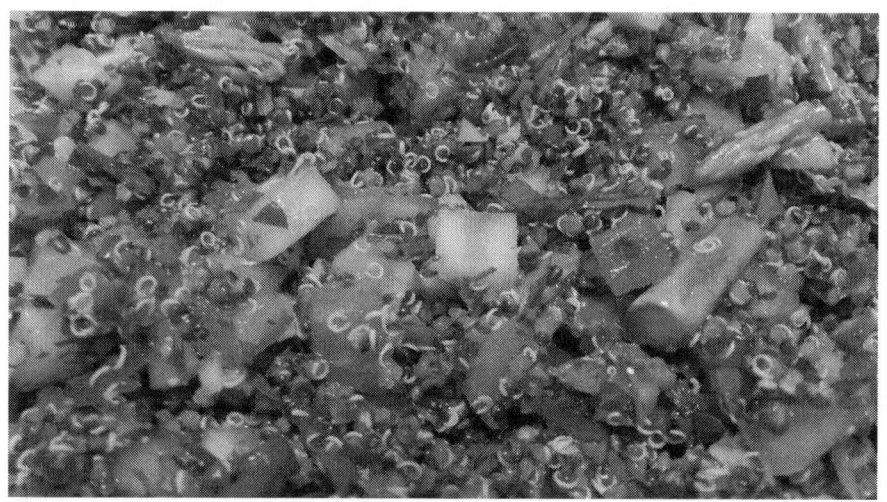

Makes 4-6 Servings

FIXINGS

¾ cup bulgur
1½ cups water
2 cups newly cleaved parsley
¾ cup cleaved scallions, white and green parts ½ red chime pepper, diced
½ green ringer pepper, diced
½ cup finely cleaved new mint
½ cup new lemon juice
½ cup extra-virgin olive oil
Ocean salt and newly ground pepper to taste
3 ready plum tomatoes, stripped, seeded, and diced 1 enormous cucumber, stripped, seeded, and diced

Bunch of greens for serving
Prepared pita wedges

METHOD

In a little pan absorb bulgur water for 30 minutes. Channel bulgur through a strainer and permit it to dry completely. Clean parsley under virus running water and press tenderly between paper towels to dry. Spot bulgur, parsley, scallions, peppers, and mint in a huge bowl.

Mix to blend well. In a different bowl whisk together lemon juice and olive oil. Season bulgur blend with salt and pepper to taste. Add lemon blend to bulgur—sufficiently just to make plate of mixed greens wet (not runny)— and hurl.
Crease in tomatoes and cucumber, at that point spread and chill. Serve on a bed of greens, with prepared pita wedges for plunging. This serving of mixed greens works out positively for toasted, herb-prepared entire wheat pita triangles.

GREEK WHITE FAVA BEAN (WITH MIXED GREENS)

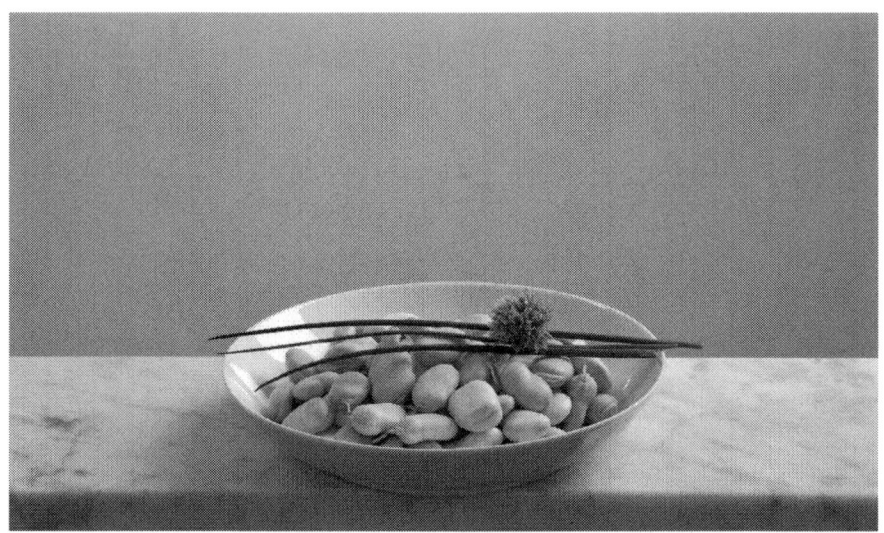

Makes 4 Servings

FIXINGS

1¼ cups dried white fava beans
2–3 new sage leaves
Salt to taste
2 cloves new garlic, finely minced
1 little onion, finely slashed
1 celery stem, finely slashed
3 tablespoons new lemon juice
½ teaspoon dried oregano
3 tablespoons extra-virgin olive oil
4½ tablespoons red wine vinegar

Newly ground pepper to taste

METHOD

Drench the beans for the time being in new (water must cover the beans by twice their volume). Toward the beginning of the day, channel beans, flush with new water, and channel a second time.

Join depleted beans and 1 quart of new water in an enormous pot; heat to the point of boiling. Include sage, spread pot, and cook for around 45 minutes. Delicately mix what's more, add salt to taste.

Keep cooking for about an additional 15 minutes, until beans are delicate however not soft. Expel from warmth and channel. Let beans cool somewhat, at that point hurl with garlic, onion, celery, lemon juice, oregano, olive oil, and vinegar. Add pepper to taste, and chill for 1 hour or more before serving.

ORANGE BROILED ASPARAGUS

Makes 6 Servings

FIXINGS

1 pound new asparagus, cut and cut into ½-inch slanting pieces
4 tablespoons extra-virgin olive oil
Salt to taste
4 tablespoons new, sweet, no-mash squeezed orange 1 tablespoon newly crushed lime juice
2 cloves finely minced garlic
Salt and newly ground pepper to taste
6 cups slashed new romaine lettuce
3 tablespoons toasted pine nuts
1 tablespoon minced new basil leaf
Newly ground Romano cheddar (discretionary)

METHOD

Hurl asparagus with 2 tablespoons of olive oil and salt to taste. Mastermind asparagus in a heating dish in a solitary layer and spot in broiler. Cook until delicate fresh, around 10 minutes. Put in a safe spot.

In a bowl, energetically whisk squeezed orange, lime juice, garlic, and staying 2 tablespoons of olive oil; add salt and pepper to taste. At the point when prepared to serve, partition lettuce into 6 servings, organize on plate of mixed greens plates, and top with asparagus.

Quickly whisk the dressing and pour over lettuce what's more, asparagus plate of mixed greens. Top with pine nuts and basil. Embellishment with a limited quantity of Romano cheddar, whenever wanted to toast pinenuts in the stove: spot the nuts in a single layer on a non-stick heating sheet.

Prepare at 375 degrees, blending once in a while, until daintily seared. Expel from broiler and permit to cool.

MEDITERRANEAN BLENDED GREENS

Makes 4-6 Servings

FIXINGS

6 cups arranged new blended greens, (for example, arugula, radicchio, infant spinach, watercress, and romaine)
1 little red onion, daintily cut and isolated into rings
20 firm cherry tomatoes, split
¼ cup cleaved pecans
¼ cup dried cranberries
Disintegrated feta cheddar (discretionary)
Newly ground pepper to taste

For Dressing:

2 tablespoons balsamic vinegar
4 tablespoons extra-virgin olive oil
1 tablespoon water
½ teaspoon squashed dried oregano
2 cloves new garlic, finely minced

METHOD

In an enormous serving of mixed greens bowl, consolidate greens, onion, tomatoes, pecans, and cranberries. Delicately hurl.

Dressing:
Join vinegar, olive oil, water, oregano, and garlic; shake well. Pour dressing over serving of mixed greens and hurl softly to cover. Topping with feta cheddar, whenever wanted, and pepper to taste.

Approx. 140 calories for every serving 2g protein, 12g all out fat, 1g immersed fat, 0 trans fat, 6g starches, 0 cholesterol, 47mg sodium, 1g fiber

NORTH AFRICAN ZUCCHINI

Makes 4 Servings

FIXINGS

1 pound firm green zucchini, daintily cut
Juice from 1 huge lemon
2 cloves new garlic, finely minced
½ teaspoon ground cumin
1 tablespoon extra-virgin olive oil
1½ tablespoons plain low-fat yogurt
Salt and newly ground pepper to taste
Finely slashed parsley for embellish
Disintegrated feta cheddar (discretionary)

METHOD

Steam zucchini until fresh delicate, approximately 2–5 minutes. Wash under virus water and channel well. In an enormous plate of mixed greens bowl, blend the lemon juice, garlic, cumin, olive oil, yogurt, and salt and pepper to taste.

Include zucchini and delicately hurl. Chill in the fridge for 45 minutes to 1 hour before serving. Enhancement with parsley furthermore, feta cheddar, whenever wanted.

GREENS WITH CHEDDAR EMBLEMS

Makes 6 Servings

FIXINGS

6 ounces delicate goat cheddar, log style
½ cup extra-virgin olive oil, separated down the middle
¼ cup plain bread morsels
2 tablespoons newly squashed garlic
Olive oil cooking splash
6 cups (approximately 16–18 ounces) blended greens, for example, escarole, red and green leaf lettuce, radicchio, and endive, washed and all around dried
1 cup split cherry tomatoes
2 tablespoons red wine vinegar

2 teaspoons Dijon mustard
Salt and newly ground pepper to taste
Finely hacked walnuts (discretionary)

METHOD

Preheat oven. Cut goat cheddar sign into 6 equivalent pieces and spot cheddar emblems in a bowl containing ¼ cup olive oil; softly wash blend. Move the oil-loaded cheddar emblems to a bowl containing a blend of bread morsels furthermore, squashed garlic.

Coat emblems on the two sides with bread scraps and garlic blend. Gently splash a heating sheet with cooking oil and spot emblems on sheet; cook until brilliant earthy colored and fresh, 1–2 minutes for each side.

Hurl greens with tomatoes, separate into 6 segments, and top each bit with a cheddar emblem. Consolidate the remaining ¼ cup olive oil, red wine vinegar, and Dijon mustard in a jug and shake to blend well.

Sprinkle blend over servings of mixed greens. Include salt and pepper to taste. Enhance with walnuts, whenever wanted, before serving.

FENNEL SALAD

Makes 4-6 Servings

FIXINGS

1 huge clove new garlic, divided
1 huge fennel bulb, meagerly cut
½ English cucumber, daintily cut
1 tablespoon minced new chives
8 huge radishes, meagerly cut
3 tablespoons extra-virgin olive oil
2½ tablespoons newly pressed lemon juice
Salt and newly ground pepper to taste
Marinated blended olives (discretionary)

METHOD

Rub within a huge bowl with garlic. Include fennel, cucumber, chives, and radishes. In a different bowl whisk together olive oil, new lemon squeeze, and salt furthermore, pepper to taste.

Pour olive oil blend over plate of mixed greens and hurl to blend. Topping with marinated olives, whenever wanted.

AVOCADO SALAD

Makes 3 Servings

FIXINGS

1 enormous ready avocado, hollowed and stripped
1 cup divided cherry tomatoes
2 tablespoons cleaved new parsley
1 little onion, finely cleaved
½ little hot pepper, finely cleaved (discretionary) 2 teaspoons new lime juice
Salt and newly ground pepper to taste

METHOD

Cut avocado into reduced down lumps. Join tomatoes, parsley, onion, hot pepper, and lime juice. Hurl well; add salt and pepper to taste. Include avocado and hurl delicately. Partition into 3 equivalent bits and serve.

TUNISIAN CARROT SALAD

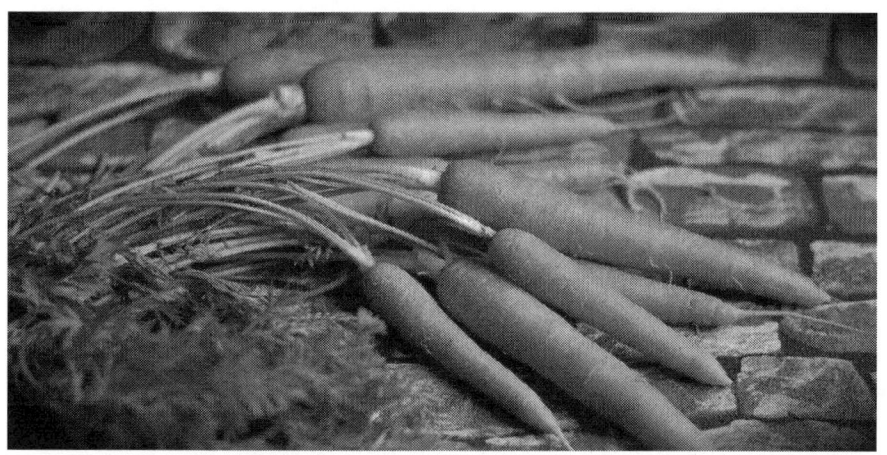

Makes 6 Servings

FIXING

10 medium carrots, stripped and cut into ½-inch-thick cuts
5 teaspoons newly minced garlic
Salt to taste
2 teaspoons caraway seed
6 tablespoons juice vinegar
¼ cup extra-virgin olive oil
1 cup disintegrated feta cheddar, separated

METHOD

20 pitted Kalamata olives, saving some for embellish In a medium poloaded up with water, cook carrots until delicate. Channel and cool under virus running water, at

that point channel again and place in a bowl.

Consolidate garlic, salt, what's more, caraway seed in a mortar and granulate until it frames an unpleasant glue, at that point beat the glue in a food processor. Add vinegar to the bowl with the carrots and blend well.

Squash the carrots. Include the garlic-caraway blend to Vinegar-carrot blend, mix well, and blend in olive oil. Include ¾ cup feta cheddar and olives and hurl once more.

Spot serving of mixed greens in a shallow bowl what's more, embellish with remaining feta cheddar and olives.

TUNISIAN TUNA SALAD

Makes 4 Servings

FIXINGS

3 huge ready tomatoes, stripped
2 medium green chime peppers, seeded and cut into slim rings
1 enormous cucumber, cut
1 sweet onion, meagerly cut and isolated into rings
2 hard-bubbled eggs, shelled and isolated into quarters

2 tablespoons new lemon juice
2 cloves new garlic, minced
2 tablespoons red wine vinegar
1 tablespoon water
1 teaspoon Dijon mustard
2 tablespoons slashed new basil
¼ cup extra-virgin olive oil
1 (12-ounce) can water-pressed white tuna fish, depleted and separated into 4 equivalent amounts
Salt and newly ground pepper to taste
Kalamata olives, cleaved, for embellish
Gap tomatoes, chime peppers, cucumber, onion, and eggs into 4 bits.

METHOD

On 4 individual serving of mixed greens platters first layer tomatoes, at that point spread with layers of pepper rings, cucumber cuts, and onion rings. Orchestrate eggs around edges of platters.

In a little bowl, whisk the lemon juice, garlic, vinegar, water, mustard, and basil together until smooth. Step by step rush in olive oil. Pour dressing over each serving of mixed greens platter.

Spot a scoop of fish on the focal point of every serving of mixed greens, and include salt and pepper to taste. Topping with escapades and olives.

CHOPPED SALAD WITH WALNUT DRESSING

Makes 6 servings

FIXINGS

3 medium ready tomatoes, seeded and hacked
1 medium cucumber, stripped, seeded, and diced
1 huge green ringer pepper, seeded and diced
5 scallions, finely hacked
1 head chunk of ice lettuce
¼ cup new spearmint leaves, finely hacked
20 pitted Kalamata dark olives

For Walnut Dressing:

2 cuts Italian bread, absorbed water, pressed dry, and disintegrated ¼ cup finely minced shelled pecans
½ teaspoon finely squashed garlic
¼ cup extra-virgin olive oil
Lemon juice, newly pressed, to taste
Salt to taste (discretionary)
Scorching pepper sauce to taste (discretionary)

METHOD

In a huge blending bowl consolidate tomatoes, cucumber, green ringer pepper, and scallions. Include Walnut Dressing and hurl altogether. Add salt to taste. Line a serving platter with lettuce leaves. Spoon plate of mixed greens blend over cleaned and isolated lettuce leaves, sprinkle with spearmint, and trimming with olives.

Serve right away.

Pecan Dressing:

In a blender or food processor include bread, pecans, and garlic and mix while gradually including olive oil. Bit by bit include lemon squeeze and beat until blend is smooth.

Include salt and hot pepper sauce to taste.

SPANISH SALAD

Makes 6 Servings

FIXINGS

1 pack (2 bundles) cleaned and cut romaine lettuce, attacked scaled down pieces
3 medium ready tomatoes, cut into ¼-inch wedges
1 enormous sweet onion, meagerly cut
1 green ringer pepper, seeded and daintily cut
1 red chime pepper, seeded and meagerly cut

¼ cup slashed and pitted marinated green olives
¼ cup hacked and pitted dark olives
¼ cup extra-virgin olive oil
3 tablespoons balsamic vinegar
Salt and newly ground pepper to taste (discretionary)

METHOD

Place a bed of romaine lettuce on 6 chilled serving of mixed greens plates. Mastermind tomatoes, onion, peppers, and olives on the lettuce on each plate. Blend olive oil and vinegar together; shower over serving of mixed greens. Include salt and pepper, whenever wanted, and serve.

COUSCOUS PARSLEY SALAD

Makes 4 Servings

FIXINGS

¼ cup couscous
¼ cup water
2 tablespoons new lemon juice
2 teaspoons extra-virgin olive oil
¼ cup finely hacked new level parsley leaves

2 tablespoons finely cleaved new mint leaves
2 teaspoons lemon get-up-and-go
2 tablespoons pine nuts
Salt and newly ground pepper to taste
1 medium ready tomato, stripped, seeded, and diced
2 heads Belgian endive, leaves for scooping
Entire wheat pita adjusts, cut into wedges and toasted until firm (discretionary)

METHOD

Consolidate couscous with water and lemon juice in a medium bowl, and let represent 60 minutes. Following 60 minutes, include olive oil, parsley, mint, lemon get-up-and-go, pine nuts, and salt and pepper to taste.

Blend well. Shape couscous blend into a hill in the focal point of a serving platter and trimming with tomato. Encompass with endive leaves or toasted pita wedges, whenever wanted. Serve at room temperature.

PASTA AND SHRIMP SALAD

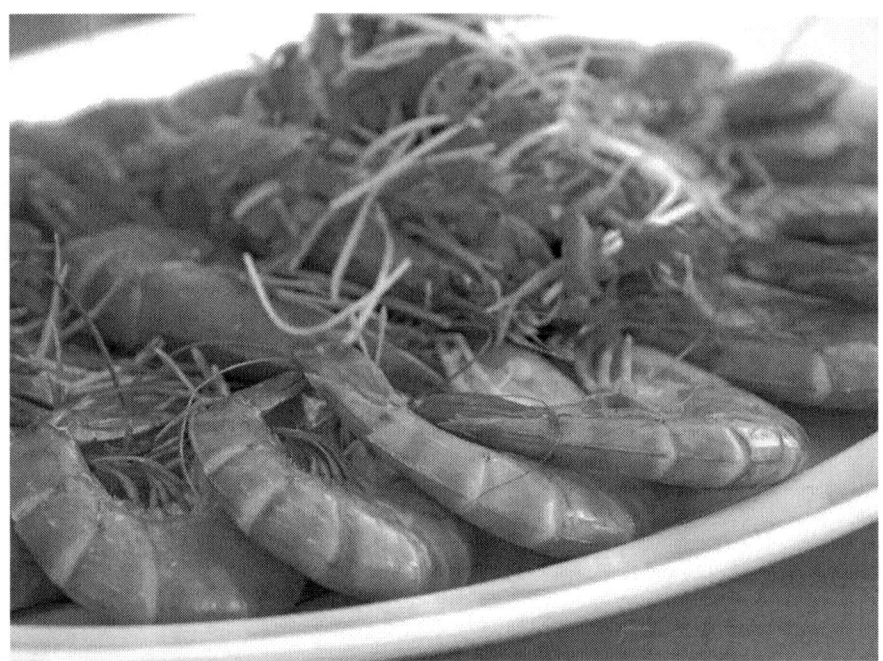

Makes 6 Servings

FIXINGS

½ pound entire wheat fettuccine
16 enormous (around 1 pound) pre-cooked shrimp
12 pitted dark olives, divided
6 cherry tomatoes, divided
½ cup diced simmered red peppers
¼ cup slashed new parsley
¼ cup slashed new basil
4 scallions, cut and cut
¼ pound feta cheddar, disintegrated

Salt and newly ground pepper to taste
Extra-virgin olive oil to sprinkle

METHOD

Fill an enormous pot with water and warmth to bubbling, include pasta, and cook until aldente. At the point when prepared, channel pasta well and move to an enormous serving bowl.

Include cooked shrimp, olives, tomatoes, peppers, parsley, basil, scallions, and feta cheddar to pasta. Hurl to blend. Include salt and pepper and shower with olive oil to daintily soak pasta; serve.

TANGERINE CRESS SALAD

Makes 6 Servings

FIXINGS

4 huge sweet tangerines
Juice from 1 new lemon
¼ cup extra-virgin olive oil
Ocean salt and newly ground pepper to taste

2 huge bundles watercress (washed, with intense stems expelled)
10 cherry tomatoes, split
16 pitted Kalamata olives

METHOD

Strip tangerines and separate segments. Evacuate any pits and press areas to get ¼ cup of juice. Put segments in a safe spot. In a huge bowl, whisk together tangerine juice, lemon juice, olive oil, and salt and pepper to taste.

Pat watercress dry with paper towels to expel any overabundance water. Include watercress, tomatoes, and olives to tangerine areas in a huge bowl and hurl with oil blend.

Serve quickly on chilled plate of mixed greens plates.

TOASTED CAPRI SALAD

Makes 4 Servings

FIXINGS

1 enormous firm ready tomato, cut into 8 slim cuts
8 meager cuts of red onion
1 (around 8-ounce) bundle of new mozzarella cheddar, cut into 8 cuts
12 pitted Kalamata olives, divided
8 entire new basil leaves, decorate for plates Aged balsamic vinegar to sprinkle
Extra-virgin olive oil to sprinkle
Ocean salt and newly ground pepper to taste
Newly slashed basil for embellish

METHOD

Preheat broiler to sear. Gap initial 4 fixings into 4 equivalent parts. Exchange fixings beginning with tomato, onion, and cheddar, and top with a couple olives to make 4 separate stacks.

Spot stacks in a broiler safe dish around 4 inches under oven, and cook for around 2–3 minutes or until cheddar mostly dissolves. Expel from stove. Spot 2 entire basil leaves on each plate and top with toasted plate of mixed greens stack.

Sprinkle limited quantity of vinegar and olive oil over each plate of mixed greens, include salt and pepper, whenever wanted, decorate with hacked basil, and serve.

ENDIVE SPINACH SALAD

Makes 6 Servings

FIXINGS

Olive oil cooking splash
½ cup hacked pecans
¼ cup extra-virgin olive oil
4 tablespoons newly hacked shallots
2 tablespoons white wine vinegar
1 tablespoon unadulterated maple syrup
Salt to taste
¼ teaspoon newly ground pepper
1 (10-ounce) pack cleaned new spinach
2 heads Belgian endive
1½ tablespoons slashed dried cranberries
¼ cup disintegrated Danish blue cheddar

METHOD

Shower a little substantial bottomed skillet with cooking oil and gently toast pecans over medium warmth. Mix continually to shield from consuming. Expel from warmth and put in a safe spot. In a little bowl, whisk together olive oil, shallots, vinegar, syrup, salt, and pepper.

Put aside to wed flavors. Spot cleaned spinach in a huge serving of mixed greens bowl. Cut endive on the corner to corner into dainty cuts with a sharp blade what's more, add to spinach.

Add cranberries and pecans to spinach, and hurl all fixings with dressing. Sprinkle plate of mixed greens with blue cheddar and serve.

CHICKPEAS AND GARDEN VEGETABLES

Makes 4 Servings

FIXINGS

2 tablespoons newly pressed lemon juice
2 cloves new garlic, finely minced
1 tablespoon new basil leaf, cut
⅛ teaspoon newly ground pepper
1 (15-ounce) can chickpeas, washed and all around depleted
2 cups coarsely hacked new broccoli
½ cup cut new carrots
1 (7½-ounce) can diced tomatoes, undrained
1 cup cubed part-skim mozzarella cheddar

METHOD

In a huge serving bowl consolidate lemon juice, garlic, basil, and ground pepper.

Mix in chickpeas, broccoli, carrots, tomatoes with juice, and mozzarella cheddar.

Hurl fixings, blending admirably. Cover and refrigerate for at any rate 4 hours.

PEPPERY WATERCRESS SALAD

Makes 4-6 Servings

FIXINGS

2 bundles (around 8 cups) watercress, washed and unpleasant stems expelled
2 teaspoons champagne vinegar
Salt and newly ground pepper to taste
2 tablespoons extra-virgin olive oil

METHOD

Permit watercress to deplete. In a little bowl, whisk together vinegar, salt and pepper, and olive oil. Spot watercress in a serving of mixed greens bowl and hurl well with olive oil blend to cover equitably.

Serve right away.

HERBED POTATO SALAD

Makes 4 Servings

FIXINGS

2 pounds red skin potatoes, cubed
14 ounces low-sodium, sans fat chicken stock
2 cloves new garlic, minced
½ cup plain low-fat yogurt
1 tablespoon cleaved new dill
1 tablespoon cleaved new oregano
2 tablespoons light mayonnaise
2 tablespoons extra-virgin olive oil
2 tablespoons white wine vinegar
Salt and newly ground pepper to taste

METHOD

In an enormous pan, include 2 cups water, potatoes, chicken stock, and garlic. Cook over medium-high warmth for around 20 minutes or until potatoes are delicate. Deplete and permit to cool.

Whisk together yogurt, dill, oregano, mayonnaise, olive oil, vinegar, and salt and pepper. Tenderly overlay potatoes into yogurt blend and chill for in any event 2 hours before serving.

WATERMELON SALAD

Makes 4 Servings

FIXINGS

2 cups cubed seedless watermelon
Salt and newly ground pepper to taste
2 cups arugula
1 cup cut cucumber, with skin on
4 ounces new feta cheddar, cut into reduced down pieces
3 tablespoons extra virgin olive oil
2 teaspoons white balsamic vinegar

METHOD

Add watermelon to an enormous plate of mixed greens bowl and sprinkle with salt and pepper to taste. Include arugula, cucumber, and feta; hurl to blend. Join olive oil and vinegar, and sprinkle over plate of mixed greens.

Prepare to cover plate of mixed greens and serve.

SUMMER PASTA SALAD

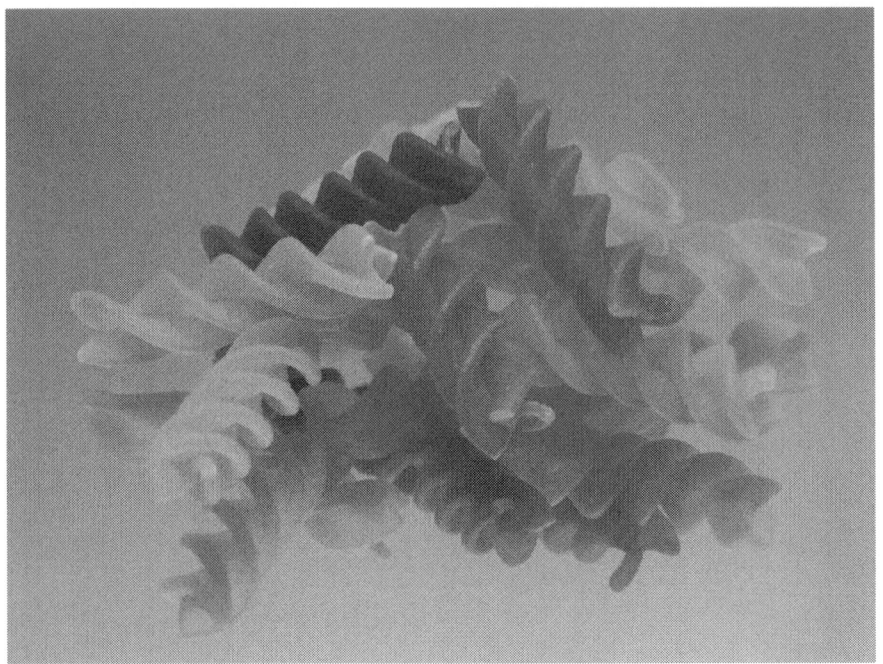

Makes 4 Servings

FIXINGS

5 ounces entire wheat Fusilli pasta
4 cups inexactly stuffed child arugula
⅓ cup sundried tomatoes, cleaved
2 tablespoons escapades, washed and depleted
2 tablespoons shaved Parmesan cheddar
Low-calorie dressing of decision

METHOD

Cook pasta according to bundle guidelines and channel. Consolidate pasta with arugula, tomatoes, and escapades. Tenderly hurl to blend.

Include Parmesan cheddar and dressing of decision.

ESCAROLE WITH ANCHOVY DRESSING

Makes 4 Servings

FIXINGS

4 cups scaled down escarole
3 scallions, cleaved
½ (6.5-ounce) can cut dark olives, all around depleted
Shaved Parmesan cheddar for embellish

For Anchovy Dressing:

2 tablespoons red wine vinegar
1 teaspoon Dijon mustard
Juice from 1 lemon
1 clove new garlic, minced
3 level anchovies, crushed
6 tablespoons extra-virgin olive oil
Salt and newly ground pepper to taste

Direction:

Tear and clean escarole, channel, and put in a safe spot.

METHOD

In a little bowl, whisk together vinegar, mustard, and lemon juice. Mix in garlic and anchovies and gradually rush in olive oil. Add salt and pepper to taste. Refrigerate to chill. In a huge plate of mixed greens bowl, consolidate escarole, scallions, and olives, hurl with chilled dressing, top with Parmesan shavings, and serve.

PEAR AND WALNUT SALAD

Makes 4 Servings

FIXINGS

2 cups low-sodium, without fat chicken stock
1 cup white grain quinoa
2 tablespoons canola oil
1 tablespoon raspberry vinaigrette
¼ cup cut new chives
Salt and newly ground pepper to taste

2 ready yet firm pears, cored and diced
½ cup toasted pecans for embellish

METHOD

In a huge pan, heat stock to a bubble. Mix in quinoa, cover and diminish to a stew, and cook until fluid is consumed, around 15–20 minutes. While quinoa stews, in a bowl whisk together canola oil, vinaigrette, chives, and salt and pepper. Add pears and hurl to cover.

Channel any overabundance staying fluid from quinoa and add quinoa to pears. Hurl to blend well. Spot pear-quinoa blend in fridge and chill for around 15 minutes. Serve cold with a sprinkling of pecans.

CRUNCHY CHICKEN AND FRUIT SALAD

Makes 4 Servings

FIXINGS

¼ cup walnuts, hacked
3 cups hacked broiled chicken, bosom meat just
1 enormous head Bibb lettuce

2 ready tangerines, stripped and segmented
2 little Granny Smith apples, cored and coarsely hacked For

Dressing:

⅓ cup light mayonnaise
1 orange, split

Salt and newly ground pepper to taste

Direction:

In a little bowl include mayonnaise. Crush juice from orange. Mix enough juice into mayonnaise until it has a dressing consistency. Add salt and pepper to taste.

METHOD

In a little skillet over low warmth, toast walnuts, mixing much of the time until brilliant earthy colored, and put in a safe spot. Separation chicken, lettuce, tangerine cuts, and apples into 4 divides.

Organize on singular plates. Include a sprinkling of toasted walnuts and sprinkle each presenting with dressing.

PEAR AND WATERCRESS SALAD

Makes 4 Servings.

FIXINGS

4 ready however firm smooth-skin pears
2 cups watercress
2 tablespoons toasted walnut parts
2 ounces disintegrated blue cheddar
¼ cup vinaigrette dressing
Juice from 1 lemon
Nectar to sprinkle

METHOD

Center every pear from the base up leaving stem flawless. In a bowl include watercress, walnuts, blue cheddar, and vinaigrette. Hurl well to cover and put in a safe spot.

Cut every pear in 4 even cuts. Brush cut sides with lemon juice. Reassemble pears into unique shape, including serving of mixed greens blend between each cut.

Sprinkle pears with nectar and serve.

MUSHROOM AND BARLEY SALAD

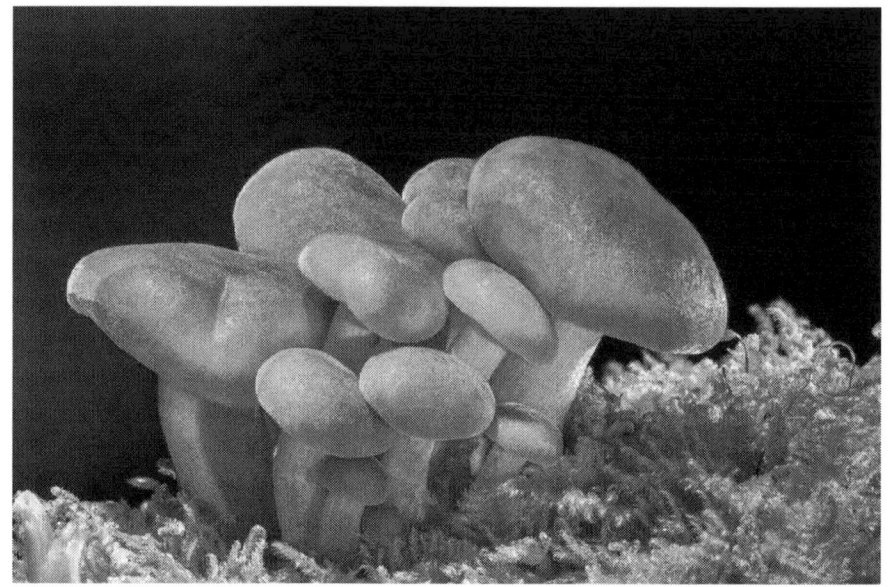

Makes 6 Servings

FIXINGS.

½ cup extra-virgin olive oil, separated
1½ pounds arranged mushrooms, split and separated
 Salt and newly ground pepper to taste
2 heads Bibb lettuce, leaves isolated
1½ cups cooked grain
½ cup toasted hacked hazelnuts
½ cup new level leaf parsley

For Dressing:

1 shallot, minced
3 tablespoons sherry vinegar, separated
½ cup low-fat sharp cream
3 tablespoons hacked new chives
3 teaspoons new thyme

Salt and newly ground pepper to taste

METHOD

Warmth 1 tablespoon olive oil in a huge skillet over medium warmth. Include half of the mushrooms and sauté until brilliant earthy colored, mixing frequently. Move to an enormous plate of mixed greens bowl.

Rehash for rest of mushrooms. Add salt and pepper to taste to mushrooms in bowl. In a similar bowl, include lettuce, grain, hazelnuts, and parsley. Include dressing, hurling to cover, and keeping in mind that serving hurl incidentally to keep on covering.

CHOPPED GARDEN SALAD

Makes 4 Servings

FIXINGS

½ head icy mass lettuce, destroyed
1 enormous carrot, cleaned and finely slashed
3 stems celery, cleaned and finely cleaved
½ little red onion, finely diced
4 enormous red radishes, slashed
½ (6.5-ounce) can cut dark ready olives, very much depleted
½ (6.5-ounce) can chickpeas, very much depleted
4 teaspoons julienne-cut sundried tomatoes in olive oil
4 tablespoons oil from the sundried tomato container
½ medium ready yet firm tomato, diced
½ enormous avocado, cut into ½-inch blocks
Salt and newly ground pepper to taste

METHOD

In an enormous serving of mixed greens bowl, join lettuce, carrot, celery, onion, radishes, dark olives, chickpeas, and sundried tomatoes. Sprinkle serving of mixed greens with the oil from sundried tomato.

Delicately prepare serving of mixed greens until very much blended. Disperse diced tomato and avocado pieces over top of serving of mixed greens, and season with salt and pepper.

Enhancement with bread garnishes, whenever wanted, and serve.

CUCUMBER SALAD

Makes 2 Servings

FIXINGS

1 enormous cucumber, daintily cut
1 little red onion, meagerly cut
Matured red wine vinegar
Salt and newly ground dark pepper to taste

METHOD

Place cucumber and onion cuts in a bowl and spread them with vinegar. Spread and chill for at any rate 1–2

2.4 MEDITERRANEAN DIET SOUPS

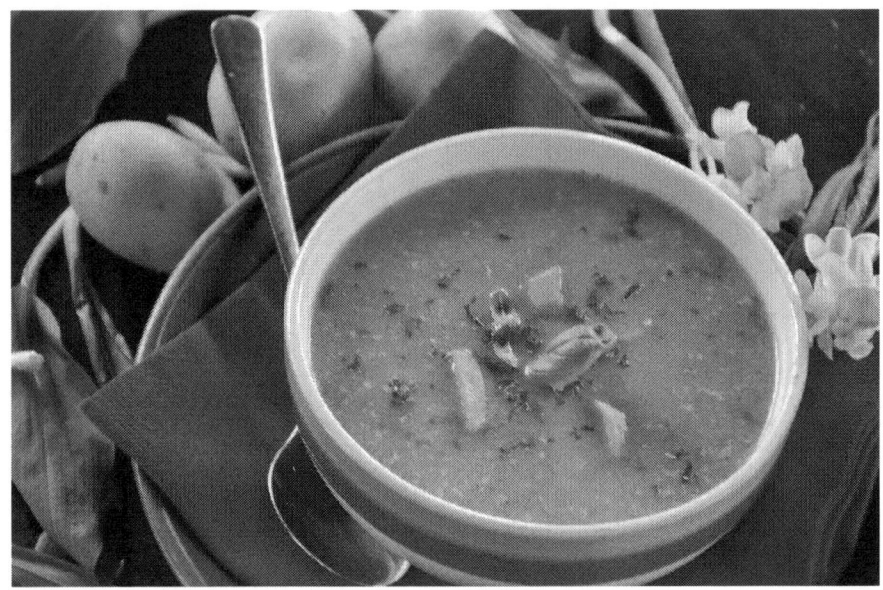

CHICKEN BROTH

Makes 6-6 1/2 Servings

FIXINGS

2 pounds skinless, bone-in chicken
2 stems celery with leaves, cut into lumps
1 enormous white onion, quartered
2 medium carrots, cut into lumps
2 cloves new garlic, diced

1 teaspoon dry Italian flavoring blend
9 cups cold water

METHOD

Put all the fixings into a huge pot and heat to the point of boiling. Utilizing an opened spoon, skim froth from the surface. Diminish warmth to a delicate stew, spread, and cook for 2 hours.

Expel chicken and put aside to cool. Strain fluid through a sifter, disposing of vegetables and seasonings. Refrigerate staying stressed stock for a few hours to chill. Prior to utilizing stock, skim fat from surface.

Refrigerated, stock can be accumulated to 3–4 days or it very well may be solidified and hidden away to 3 months. Cooled chicken can be deboned and utilized for different plans.

GREEN GARDEN SOUP

Makes 6 Servings

FIXINGS

4 tablespoons trans fat–free canola/olive oil spread
1 white onion, slashed
4 cloves new garlic, minced
1 enormous leek, meagerly cut white parts and cut green parts, keep separate
8 ounces new brussels grows, cut
5 ounces new green beans, meagerly cut
5 cups low-sodium, sans fat vegetable stock
1½ cups solidified peas, defrosted
1 tablespoon newly crushed lemon juice
1 teaspoon ground coriander
1 cup low-fat milk
4 teaspoons generally useful flour
Salt and newly ground pepper to taste

METHOD

In a huge skillet, liquefy canola/olive oil spread over low warmth. Include onion and garlic and cook until delicate and fragrant, yet don't brown. Include the green pieces of the leek, brussels sprouts, and green beans to the skillet. Add stock and heat to the point of boiling.

Lessen warmth and let stew for 10 minutes. Include peas, lemon juice, and coriander and keep on letting stew for 10–15 minutes more or until vegetables are delicate.

Expel vegetable blend from warmth and permit to cool somewhat, at that point move to a blender or food processor and procedure until smooth. Come back to a pot and include white pieces of leek.

Heat to the point of boiling over medium-high warmth, at that point diminish to a stew for around 5 minutes, and diminish again to keep warm. In a separate little bowl, whisk together milk and flour until smooth.

Include flour blend to soup, mixing to join, and add salt and pepper to taste. Serve with a dispersing of bread garnishes on top, whenever wanted.

LEMONY CHICKEN AND ORZO SOUP

Makes 4 Servings

FIXINGS

1 tablespoon olive oil
½ cup hacked white onion
½ cup hacked celery
6 cups low-sodium, without fat chicken stock
½ cup cut carrot
12 ounces skinless, boneless chicken bosoms
Salt and newly ground pepper to taste
½ cup orzo
¼ cup hacked new dill
Lemon parts to press

METHOD

In a huge pot, heat olive oil over medium warmth. Include onion and celery and cook until vegetables are delicate. Include chicken stock, carrot, chicken, and salt and pepper to taste.

Heat to the point of boiling, at that point decrease warmth to a stew, and cook for approximately 20 minutes until chicken is cooked. Expel chicken from stock, permit to cool, at that point shred chicken into scaled down pieces and put in a safe spot.

Keep stock pot secured and on extremely low warmth to keep warm while destroying chicken. Include orzo to stock, return stock to a bubble, and cook for around 8 minutes. Expel pot from heat, add chicken and dill to stock, and present with a solid crush of new lemon juice.

CHILLED AVOCADO SOUP

Makes 4-6 Servings

FIXINGS

3 medium ready avocados, split, seeded, stripped, and slice to lumps
½ cucumber, stripped and hacked
½ cup hacked white onion
¼ cup finely diced carrot
2 cloves new garlic, minced
2 cups low-sodium, without fat chicken stock, isolated Hot red pepper sauce to taste
Salt and newly ground pepper to taste
Paprika to sprinkle
Sharp cream to decorate(Low Fat , optional)

METHOD

Chill 4–6 soup bowls. In a food processor or blender, consolidate avocados, cucumber, onion, carrot, garlic, and 1 cup stock, process until practically smooth. Include remaining stock, hot sauce, and salt and pepper to taste, and procedure once more until practically smooth.

Fill chilled bowls, spread tops, and chill for at any rate 1 or on the other hand more hours. To serve, expel chilled bowls and sprinkle each presenting with paprika. Include cuts of avocado and a dab of acrid cream, whenever wanted. Serve chilled.

POTATO-BROCCOLI SOUP WITH GREENS

Makes 4 Servings

FIXINGS

3 medium red-gold potatoes, hacked
2 cloves new garlic, minced
2 cups low-sodium, without fat chicken stock
3 cups new broccoli florets
3 scallions, cut
2 cups 2% milk

3 tablespoons generally useful flour
2 cups smoked Gouda cheddar, destroyed + more for embellish
Salt and newly ground pepper to taste
2 cups coarsely torn escarole departs, washed and depleted
1 cup peppered prepared bread garnishes for embellish.

METHOD

In an enormous pot, join potatoes, garlic, and stock. Heat to the point of boiling, at that point decrease heat, and let stew revealed until potatoes begin to mollify. With a substantial fork, marginally crush potatoes.

Include broccoli, scallions, and milk, and warmth to a stew until florets are fresh delicate. Decrease warmth to low, at that point include flour and Gouda cheddar, delicately mixing until cheddar melts and sauce is thickened. Season with salt and pepper to taste.

Partition soup into 4 divides. Top each presenting with escarole, extra cheddar, and a dissipating of bread garnishes, and serve.

VEGETABLE AND TORTELLINI SOUP

Makes 8-10 Servings

FIXINGS

1 huge white onion, hacked
4 cloves new garlic, hacked
3 celery stems, hacked
2 tablespoons olive oil
32 ounces low-sodium, without fat chicken stock 1 cup solidified corn
1 cup hacked carrot
1 cup solidified cut green beans
1 cup diced crude potato
1 teaspoon dried sweet basil
1 teaspoon dried thyme
1 teaspoon minced chives
2 (14.5-ounce) jars diced tomatoes, undrained
3 cups new chicken-filled tortellini Shredded without fat or low-fat cheddar (discretionary)

METHOD

In a huge pot, sauté onion, garlic, celery, also, olive oil until delicate and fragrant. Include stock, corn, carrot, beans, potato, basil, thyme, and chives. Heat to the point of boiling. Decrease warmth, spread, and let stew for around 15 minutes or until vegetables are delicate.

Include tomatoes also, tortellini and let stew revealed for an additional 5 minutes or until warmed through. Serve hot with a sprinkling cheddar and a couple dried up bread garnishes, whenever wanted.

OYSTER STEW

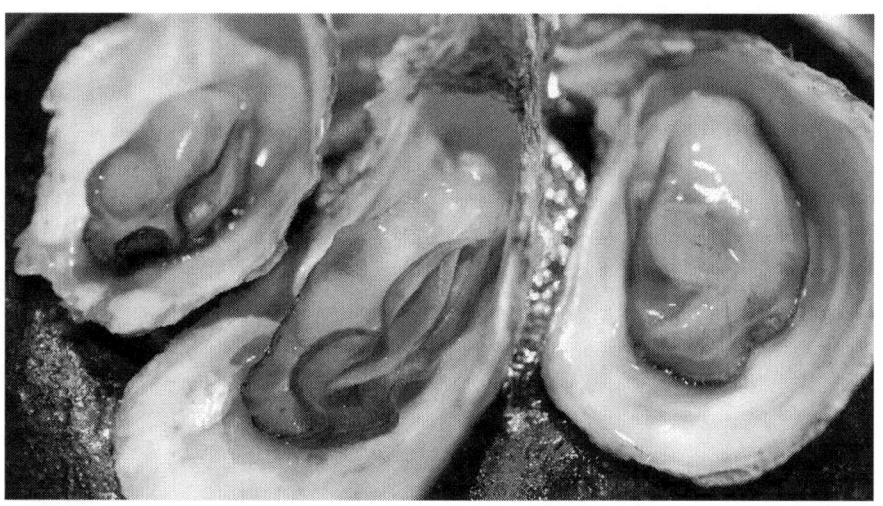

Makes 4-6 Servings

2 pints new shucked clams (around 32 ounces), undrained
4 tablespoons trans fat–free canola/olive oil spread
1 cup finely slashed celery
6 tablespoons minced shallots
3 (12-ounce) jars low-fat 2% vanished milk

Salt and newly ground pepper to taste
2 portions of cayenne pepper
Bread squares, toasted

METHOD

Channel fluid from the clams, saving the fluid. Strain the fluid through a wire sifter to evacuate any coarseness or sand. In a huge overwhelming pot, soften canola/olive oil spread over medium warmth.

Diminish warmth to a stew and include shellfish, celery, what's more, shallots. Let stew tenderly for around 4 minutes until edges of clams start to twist. While shellfish are stewing, heat milk and clam fluid in a different container over low warmth until warm.

At the point when warmed, add milk blend to clams, tenderly mixing. Add salt and pepper to taste and cayenne pepper.

Serve soup warm in warmed soup bowls with toasted bread squares.

EGGPLANT SOUP

Makes 2 Servings

FIXINGS

3 tablespoons olive oil
1 little eggplant, split and cut daintily (around 2 cups)
½ cup hacked white onion
2 cloves new garlic, minced
1 (14-ounce) can low-sodium tomato and basil pasta sauce
2 cups low sodium, without fat chicken stock
½ cup squashed decreased fat mozzarella cheddar
2 tablespoons Italian bread pieces
2 tablespoons newly ground
Parmesan cheddar for embellish Crusty bread

METHOD

In a huge non-stick dish, heat olive oil over medium-high warmth and cook eggplant for around 5 minutes, mixing every so often. Include onion and garlic and keep cooking until eggplant is brilliant earthy colored.

Include sauce and stock, bring to a bubble, at that point decrease warmth to a stew, and keep on cooking until soup thickens. Warmth stove to sear. Line a treat sheet with tin foil and spot 2 stove safe container bowls on sheet.

Gap soup into the two dishes, top with mozzarella cheddar, bread morsels, and a sprinkling of Parmesan cheddar. Cook for around 2–3 minutes or then again until cheddar is liquefied and brilliant. Serve hot with lumps of dried up bread, if wanted.

SPINACH TORTELLINI SOUP

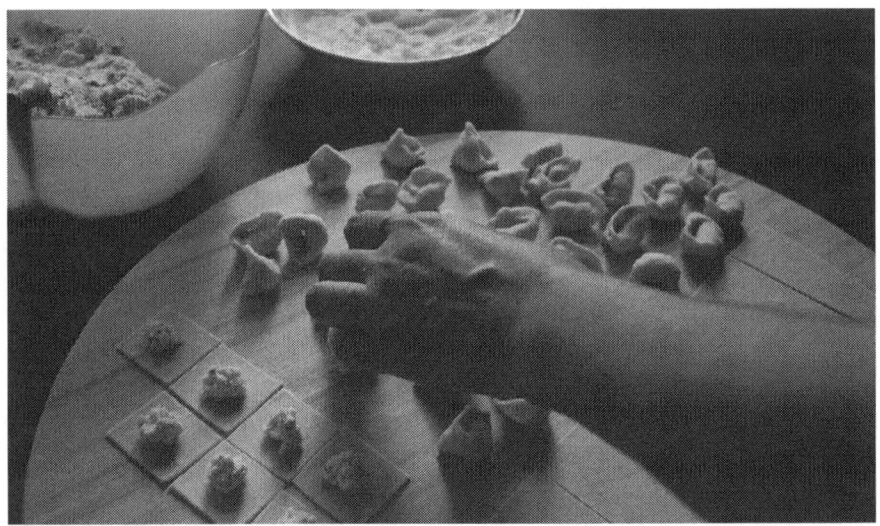

Makes 4 Servings

4 cups low-sodium, sans fat chicken stock
2 cloves new garlic, minced
4 scallions, cleaved
¼ teaspoon ground pepper
5 ounces new cheddar filled tortellini

2 cups coarsely cleaved new spinach leaves

METHOD

Heat stock in a pot and include garlic, scallions, and pepper. Heat to the point of boiling, at that point diminish to medium heat.

Include tortellini and cook for 10 minutes. Include spinach and cook for an extra 5 minutes or until pasta is delicate. Move to 4 dishes and serve with a sprinkle of Parmesan cheddar, whenever wanted.

RED CLAM CHOWDER

Makes 8-10 Servings

FIXINGS.

3 enormous stems celery, hacked
1 enormous white onion, hacked
4 (8-ounce) containers shellfish juice
4 cloves new garlic, hacked
Creole flavoring to taste
Tabasco sauce to taste
¼ cup Worcestershire sauce

¼ cup newly pressed lemon juice
3–4 cups water
1½ (14.5-ounce) jars squashed tomatoes
6 cups crude diced potatoes
4 (10-ounce) jars whole baby mollusks
Dry bread

METHOD

Consolidate all fixings, with the exception of shellfishes, hot sauce, and bread, in a huge pot. Bring to a low stew, spread, and cook for 25–30 minutes. Include shellfishes andkeep on cooking on a low stew for another 15–20 minutes. Serve hot with hot sauce, whenever wanted, and dry bread.

VEGETABLE STEW (CHILLY)

Makes 4 Servings

FIXINGS

4 cups new cauliflower florets 2 teaspoons curry powder
½ teaspoon cumin
1 (14.5-ounce) can red hot simmered diced tomatoes, undrained

2 cloves new garlic, finely minced
1 tablespoon finely cleaved Serrano bean stew pepper
1 (15-ounce) can chickpeas, depleted
¾ cup strong pressed canned pumpkin squash
¾ cup water
Salt and newly ground pepper to taste 1 cup solidified infant peas
1 cup solidified corn

METHOD

Couscous or earthy colored rice, cooked Place cauliflower florets in a pot and spread halfway with water. Heat to the point of boiling, spread, and steam until florets are practically delicate. Expel from heat, channel well, and cut enormous florets into littler sizes.

Put in a safe spot. In an enormous, non-stick skillet over medium warmth, include curry powder and cumin and warmth until fragrant. Include tomatoes with juices, garlic, stew pepper, chickpeas, pumpkin, and water.

Heat to the point of boiling, at that point decrease warmth to a stew. Include florets and salt and pepper to taste and let stew for around 15 minutes. Include peas and corn and let stew for 5 minutes longer. Expel from warmth and serve over cooked couscous or earthy colored rice.

CAULIFLOWER SOUP

Makes 6 Servings

FIXINGS

2 tablespoons olive oil
1 huge yellow onion, coarsely slashed
2 teaspoons finely cleaved new garlic
6 cups new cauliflower florets (around 1 huge head)
½ cup slashed carrot
½ cup hacked celery
1 little jalapeño pepper, seeds expelled and diced
3½ cups low-sodium, fat free chicken stock
1 (14.5-ounce) can diced tomatoes 1 inlet leaf
½ teaspoon ground cumin
Salt and newly ground pepper to taste

METHOD

Disintegrated feta cheddar for embellish Heat olive oil in an enormous pot over medium heat, include onion and garlic, and sauté until delicate. Include cauliflower florets, carrot, celery, and jalapeño. Cook until florets start to brown. Include stock, tomatoes, sound leaf, cumin, and salt and pepper, and heat to the point of boiling.

Diminish warmth to low and cook for 20–25 minutes, mixing at times, until cauliflower is delicate. Expel from heat, dispose of sound leaf, and present with bread garnishes, whenever wanted, and feta cheddar.

TOMATO TORTELLINI SOUP

Makes 8 Servings

FIXINGS

1 tablespoon olive oil
1 white onion, slashed
½ teaspoon squashed intensely hot pepper drops
2 teaspoons hacked new garlic
2 cups low-sodium, sans fat chicken stock
1 cup water
2 teaspoons hamburger bouillon base
1 (14.5-ounce) can diced low-sodium tomatoes with basil and garlic
1 (15- ounce) can low-sodium pureed tomatoes
1 tablespoon dry Italian flavoring blend
Salt and newly ground pepper to taste
1 (16-ounce) pack cheddar
tortellini
Crusty bread

METHOD

In an enormous skillet over medium warmth, include olive oil, onion, hot pepper drops, furthermore, garlic. Sauté until onion and garlic are delicate. Move to an enormous soup pot.

Include stock, water, and hamburger base to the pot, and heat to the point of boiling, at that point decrease warmth to a stew. Include tomatoes, pureed tomatoes, Italian flavoring, and salt and pepper to taste. Let stew for 15 minutes, at that point include tortellini, and let stew for another 5 minutes or until tortellini is delicate.

Serve while hot with hard bread.

STRACCIATELLA (ITALIAN EGG DROP SOUP)

Makes 4 Servings

FIXINGS

6 cups low-sodium, sans fat chicken stock
2 tablespoons minced new garlic
8 cups slashed escarole, cut into reduced down pieces
¾ cup fluid eggs
⅓ cup newly ground Parmesan cheddar Pinch of newly

ground nutmeg
2 tablespoons newly crushed lemon juice
Salt and newly ground pepper to taste
Extra-virgin olive oil to shower
Scant sum newly ground
Parmesan cheddar

METHOD

Heat chicken stock and garlic in a huge pot over medium warmth. Cover and bring to a stew, at that point include escarole and cook until delicate, around 5 minutes. Gradually include fluid eggs. As they cement, break into pieces.

Include Parmesan cheddar and nutmeg, mixing soup delicately. Decrease warmth to medium-low and cook for approximately 2–3 minutes, at that point include lemon squeeze and salt and pepper to taste.

Serve in bowls with a shower of olive oil and a sprinkle of Parmesan cheddar.

LENTIL SOUP

Makes 6-8 Servings

FIXINGS

4 cups low-sodium, sans fat chicken stock

4 cups water
1 cup split earthy colored lentils, flushed and depleted
Salt and newly ground pepper to taste
2 teaspoons ground cumin
¼ cup extra-virgin olive oil
2 medium yellow onions, finely slashed
4 enormous cloves new garlic, finely slashed
2 ounces ditalini pasta
1 enormous firm ready tomato, seeded and cut into lumps
10 ounces new escarole, washed and slashed
1 cup finely cleaved new parsley
½ cup new lemon juice

METHOD

In an enormous pot include chicken stock and water, and heat to the point of boiling. Include lentils, salt and pepper, and cumin, diminish warmth to medium, and cook until lentils are delicate.

Don't overcook; beans ought to be delicate however firm. While lentils are cooking, include olive oil to a skillet and sauté onions and garlic until brilliant earthy colored. Mix blend regularly to forestall consuming; when seared, put in a safe spot.

At the point when lentils are practically delicate, include pasta and cook until both are delicate yet not soft. Decrease warmth to a low stew, and include garlic blend, tomato, escarole, parsley, and lemon juice. Stew until escarole is cooked.

Serve embellished with a limited quantity of Parmesan cheddar, whenever wanted.

MEDITERRANEAN CHICKPEA SOUP

Makes 6 Servings

FIXINGS

2 cups water
4 cups low-sodium, without fat chicken stock
4 cups canned chickpeas, washed with new water and depleted
1 tablespoon extra-virgin olive oil
1 huge onion, hacked
4–5 cloves new garlic, minced
1 medium green chime pepper, cleaved
1 teaspoon cayenne
2 teaspoons dried sage
2 teaspoons dried rosemary
1 teaspoon ground cinnamon

Salt and newly ground pepper to taste
2 tablespoons finely hacked new parsley for embellish

METHOD

In a huge pot consolidate water, stock, chickpeas, olive oil, onion, garlic, green chime pepper, cayenne, sage, rosemary, and cinnamon. Carry blend to bubble over medium warmth, lower temperature, and stew for 20 minutes, revealed. Add salt and pepper to taste.

Embellishment with feta cheddar, and parsley if you please.

GARDEN GAZPACHO

Makes 4 Servings

FIXINGS

4 cups slashed ready stripped tomatoes
4 cloves new garlic, cleaved
½ red onion, slashed
1 green ringer pepper, seeded and diced
¼ cup extra-virgin olive oil
2 tablespoons red wine vinegar
2 cuts stale French sourdough bread

½ cup canned tomato juice
½ teaspoon cumin
½ little hot pepper, finely slashed
1 tablespoon cleaved new basil Salt and
newly ground pepper to taste
¼ cup green ringer peppers and cucumbers for decorate,

METHOD

In a food processor or blender, include tomatoes, garlic, onion, and green pepper. Mix until pureed. Include olive oil and vinegar, mix around 1 moment to blend. Absorb bread tomato juice, at that point add drenched bread blend to blender.

Include cumin, hot peppers, what's more, basil. Mix for 2–3 minutes to blend well. Change with salt and pepper to taste. Chill for a few hours. Serve very chilled, decorated with diced green peppers and cucumber.

Whenever wanted, include bread garnishes and a bit of sharp cream or yogurt.

CRISP TOMATO SOUP

Makes 4 Servings

FIXINGS

10 medium ready tomatoes
½ tablespoon extra-virgin olive oil
4–5 cloves new garlic, minced
2 tablespoons cleaved onion
2 cups low-sodium, without fat chicken stock
2 teaspoons low-calorie preparing sugar
½ teaspoon cleaved new basil
Salt and newly ground pepper to taste
2 cucumbers, diced (discretionary)

METHOD

In a huge pot of bubbling water, plunge tomatoes for 30 seconds, at that point promptly place tomatoes in chilly water. Permit to sit until they can be taken care of. Skin tomatoes with a paring blade, cut down the middle across, and expel seeds.

Center and afterward cut into quarter pieces. In a blender or food processor, process tomatoes until pureed. In a skillet, heat olive oil and sauté garlic and onion until delicate. Expel from heat.

In a huge bowl, consolidate pureed tomatoes, sautéed onion blend, chicken stock, sugar, basil, and salt and pepper, mixing to blend fixings together. Refrigerate soup for 4–6 hours until all around chilled. Trimming with, cucumbers, if you want.

ITALIAN MINESTRONE SOUP WITH PESTO

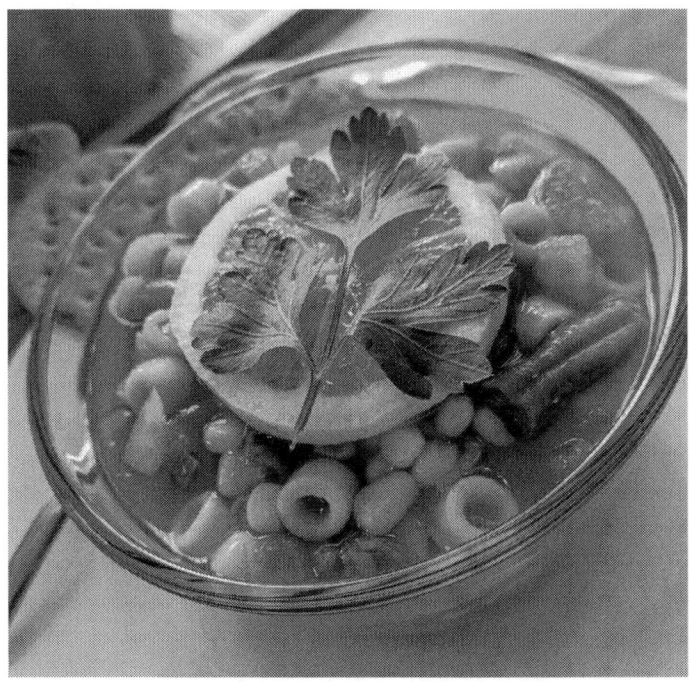

Makes 6-8 Servings

FIXINGS

1 cup dried cannellini beans
4 cups low-sodium, without fat chicken stock
4 cups water
2 medium white potatoes, stripped and diced
2 ounces ditalini pasta
2 huge carrots, cleaved
3 stems celery, cleaved
½ cup cleaved white onion
2 cloves new garlic, minced
1 cup tomato juice
3 plum tomatoes, hacked
1 huge zucchini, slashed
Cheddar(optinal)

For pesto:

1 cup new basil leaves
1 teaspoon disintegrated dried basil leaves
4 cloves new garlic, finely minced
3 tablespoons extra-virgin olive oil
½ cup ground Parmesan cheddar
Salt and newly ground pepper to taste

METHOD

Rinse dried cannellini beans and place in a huge secured pot. Include chicken stock and water and heat to the point of boiling. Reveal pot, diminish warmth, and stew until beans are delicate; around 1 hour.

Include potatoes, pasta, carrots, celery, onion, garlic, and tomato juice. Return blend to a bubble, at that point lessen warmth and stew revealed for 10 minutes. Include tomato and zucchini and stew until all are delicate.

Procedure pesto fixings in a food processor or blender until finely slashed. Expel soup from warmth and mix in pesto blend, and serve decorated with cheddar, whenever wanted.

2.5 MEDITERRANEAN DIETMAIN DISHES

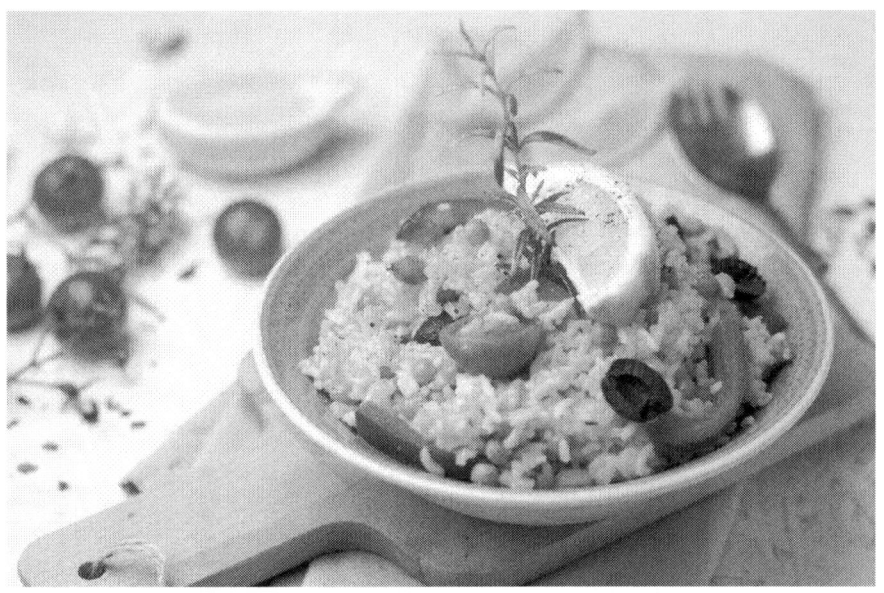

RICE-STUFFED GRAPE LEAVES

Makes 8-12 Portions(3-4 vine leaves each)

Stuffed grape leaves are equal with home, family, and occasions in many pieces of the Mediterranean. Those sold in glass containers make great substitutes. Absorb the jostled assortment bubbling water before utilizing to evacuate the briny taste.

FIXINGS

½ pound (225 g) new grape vine leaves or

1 container (8 ounces, or 225 g) saved vine leaves, depleted
1 cup (195 g) medium-grain white rice
1/3 cup (5 g) new cilantro, finely cleaved
1/3 cup (20 g) new parsley, finely cleaved
1/3 cup (16 g) new dill, finely cleaved
1/3 cup (32 g) new mint, finely cleaved
1 cup (226 g) no-sodium-included canned or boxed, cleaved or diced tomatoes, partitioned
1 medium yellow onion, ground (about ½ cup, or 80 g)
¼ cup (60 ml) extra-virgin olive oil
1 teaspoon genuine salt
1 teaspoon ground coriander
1 teaspoon cumin
Squeeze newly ground dark pepper
Squeeze bean stew powder
2 lemons, cut
1 cup Greek yogurt

METHOD

On the off chance that utilizing saved vine leaves, place them in an enormous bowl. Spread with bubbling water and let represent 10 minutes, at that point channel. Mix all the ingredients (rice, parsley, cilantro, dill, mint, 170 g of the tomatoes, onion, coriander, cumin, pepper, olive oil, salt, and bean stew powder). Spot 1 leaf on a work surface, vein side up.

Cut the abundance bit of stem from the base of each leaf.

Spot 1 tablespoon (15 g) of filling into the center of each leaf. Shape the filling to look like the width of a pencil over the width of the leaf. Roll the leaf up, beginning at the base.

Take care of the sides of the leaf as you go, making an envelope. Shun rolling the leaves too firmly or on the other hand they will tear as the rice cooks and grows inside. Proceed with the remaining leaves. Spot the stuffed vine leaves, crease side down, close to one another in a overwhelming pot.

The stuffed leaves ought to be contacting each other and fit into the dish with no spaces. Rehash a second layer on top, if essential. Spot a plate topsy turvy on top of vine leaves in the pot to shield them from rising. Pour bubbling water over the stuffed vine leaves until they are nearly, yet not totally, secured. Include the remaining ¼ cup (56 g) tomatoes and extra salt and pepper to taste, if important, to the dish.

Spread the skillet and stew on low warmth until the rice is totally cooked moreover, the leaves are sensitive, around 1 to 1½ hours. Serve warm with lemon cuts and yogurt

POTATOES WITH GARLIC, OLIVE OIL, AND CHILED PEPPER

Makes 4 Servings

This heavenly side dish is a dietary powerhouse! Potatoes contain cancer prevention agents and phytochemicals that fortify the safe framework, lower aggravation, and forestall tumor development.

FIXINGS

4 medium Yukon gold potatoes, cleaved into scaled down pieces
4 tablespoons (60 ml) extra-virgin olive oil, partitioned
4 cloves garlic, finely cleaved
Squashed red chile pepper
Ocean salt or salt
Newly ground pepper to taste
½ pound (225 g) new kale, flushed with stems and intense ribs disposed of, at that point generally cleaved

METHOD

Spot the potatoes on a heating sheet and consolidate them with 2 tablespoons (30 ml) of oil, garlic, squashed red chile pepper, salt, what's more, pepper, and prepare for 15 to 20 minutes, until brilliant and delicate. The broiler must be to 450°F (230°C).

In an enormous bowl, hurl the kale with the staying 2 tablespoons (30 ml) of oil alongside salt and pepper to taste. At the point when the potatoes have cooked, expel from the stove and disperse the kale on them. Come back to the stove and dish for an additional 10 minutes, or until kale is fresh. Serve hot

SPANISH BRAVAS-STYLE POTATOES

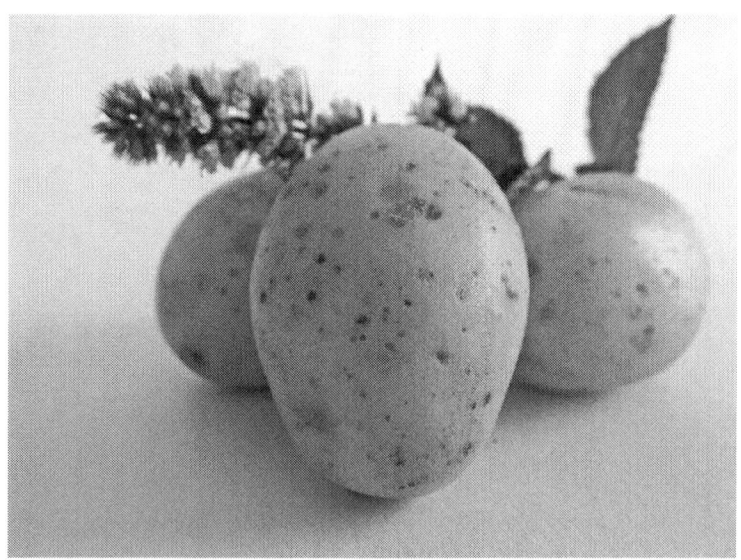

Makes 4 Servings

Bravas potatoes are a Spanish exemplary. They are arranged

distinctively in different districts in Spain.

FIXINGS

1 huge plum tomato, split and seeded
2 huge Reddish brown potatoes, stripped and cut into 1-inch (2.5 cm) 3D shapes
Unadulterated olive oil
2 cloves garlic, finely cleaved
1 tablespoon (7 g) smoked paprika
½ cup (115 g) great quality or custom made mayonnaise
 hot pepper sauce
1 tablespoon (15 ml) matured sherry vinegar
Grungy ocean salt or salt
Newly ground dark pepper
Level leaf parsley leaves

METHOD

Preheat the stove to 430°F (220°C). Broil the tomato parts on a heating sheet until delicate, 15 to 20 minutes. Expel and cool. Decrease the stove to 375°F (190°C). Spot a heating sheet in the broiler. Fill a medium pot 75% full with water.

Include the potato 3D squares and a touch of salt. Heat to the point of boiling, revealed, over high warmth. Decrease warmth to medium, and cook until simply fork-delicate, 5 to 10 minutes. Channel. Warmth 1 tablespoon (15 ml) of oil in a little griddle over medium warmth. Include the garlic and cook until it discharges its fragrance, around 3 minutes. Include the paprika and cook for 30 seconds.

Let cool marginally. Join the garlic and oil blend, mayonnaise, tomato parts, hot pepper sauce, and vinegar in a food processor and procedure until smooth. Season with salt and pepper, to taste. Put in a safe spot. Warmth 2 inches (5 cm) of unadulterated olive oil in a huge high-sided, heavy bottomed skillet until it starts to gleam, or arrives at 300°F (150°C).

Cautiously lower in half of the potatoes, and cook until brilliant earthy colored on all sides. Expel the potatoes to a paper towel–lined plate for a second to channel the overabundance oil, and season with salt and pepper. Rehash with the remaining potatoes.

Cautiously expel the hot preparing sheet from the broiler, put the potatoes on the container in an even layer and prepare until fresh, about 10 minutes. Taste, and modify seasonings if essential. Move to a platter and topping with a sprinkle of the aioli and the parsley leaves.

Serve hot.

CITRUSY SALMON WITH FENNEL CREA

Makes 4 Servings

The sweet citrus flavors consolidate with the rich, sleek surfaces in the salmon for an energizing dish that appears to be too debauched to possibly be beneficial for you. Fennel and yogurt are two famous Mediterranean fixings that are as idealistic as they are tasty.

FIXINGS

2 tablespoons (30 ml) extra-virgin olive oil
¼ cup (60 ml) squeezed orange
½ teaspoon grungy ocean salt or salt
Newly ground pepper
4 salmon filets (4 ounces, or 115 g, each), skin-on
1 fennel bulb, daintily cut (save fronds)
½ sweet onion, daintily cut
1 cup (230 g) plain Greek yogurt
2 oranges, 1 zested, 1 daintily cut

METHOD

Whisk the olive oil, squeezed orange, salt, and pepper together until emulsified. Spot the salmon filets in a glass preparing dish and pour marinade over the top. Permit to marinate for 60 minutes. Preheat the stove (400°F, 200°C). Spread fennel and onion around the sides of the salmon, and spread the preparing dish with aluminum foil.

Prepare until the fish pieces effectively with a fork also, is misty in shading, 20 to 25 minutes. While the fish is preparing, consolidate the Greek yogurt with 2 tablespoons (6 g) fennel fronds, finely hacked, and orange get-up-and-go. Expel the fish from stove and spot on a serving plate.

Dab each with about ¼ of yogurt blend and enhancement with orange cuts.

YEMISTO KALAMARI

Makes 4 Servings

FIXINGS

2 tablespoons (30 ml) extra-virgin olive oil, isolated
1 little yellow onion, finely slashed
1 pound (455 g) new spinach
¼ cup (50 g) short-grain rice
2 tablespoons (8 g) newly slashed parsley
2 tablespoons (15 g) newly slashed dill
1 teaspoon foul ocean salt or salt
Newly ground pepper
Run of squashed red bean stew chips

1 pound (455 g) infant squid, arms expelled, and cleaned
2 cups (475 ml) Vegetable or Fish Stock

METHOD

Warmth 1 tablespoon (15 ml) of olive oil in an enormous, wide skillet over medium heat. Include the onion and sauté until brilliant, around 5 minutes. Include the spinach, rice, parsley, dill, salt, pepper, and red bean stew pieces and cook for 1 moment.

Take the blend off the warmth and permit to cool somewhat. Stuff the calamari seventy five percent of the route full with stuffing.

Warmth the staying olive oil in a huge griddle over medium warmth. Earthy colored the calamari on all sides. Include the stock, spread, and stew on low until cooked through, 15 to 20 minutes, or until the rice is delicate to the chomp and the calamari are cooked through.

Serve warm.

CITRUSY SCALLOPS

Makes 4 Servings

This delightful and great dish can be cooked in minutes and filled in as a canapé or principle course. These scallops additionally taste extraordinary when prepared into a serving of mixed greens or pasta, rice, and other grain-based dishes

FIXINGS

Squeeze and get-up-and-go of 2 lemons
¼ cup (60 ml) extra-virgin olive oil
Grungy ocean salt or salt, to taste
Newly ground dark pepper, to taste
1 clove garlic
1½ pounds (650 g) dry scallops

METHOD

In a huge shallow bowl or preparing dish, consolidate the lemon squeeze and pizzazz, olive oil, salt, pepper, and garlic. Blend well to consolidate. Add the; cover and refrigerate 1 hour. Warmth a huge skillet over medium-high warmth. Channel the scallops and spot them in skillet. Cook 5 minutes for every side, until cooked through.

ROSEMARY SHRIMP OVER POLENTA

Think about this formula as the Mediterranean cousin of shrimp and corn meal. The flavorful, streak sautéed shrimp taste extraordinary

FIXINGS

¼ cup (60 ml) extra-virgin olive oil
2 cloves garlic, minced
1½ pounds (680 g) prawns or large shrimp, stripped and deveined
2 teaspoons newly hacked rosemary
Run of squashed red stew drops
½ teaspoon legitimate salt
¼ teaspoon newly ground dark pepper
3 cups cooked polenta (see page 182)

METHOD

Warmth the olive oil in a skillet. Include the garlic also, mix. Include the prawns or shrimp, rosemary, stew pieces, salt, and pepper. Cook, revealed, for around 2 minutes for each side, or until prawns or shrimp turn pink.

Spoon the polenta onto a serving platter equally, and level with the rear of a spoon. Spot prawns or shrimp on the highest point of the plate and serve right away.

SWORDFISH BUNDLES

Makes 4 Servings

Swordfish is one of the most conventional fish in the southern Italian eating routine.

FIXINGS

4 tablespoons (60 ml) extra-virgin olive oil, isolated
2 cloves garlic, minced
1 cup (226 g) slashed boxed tomatoes, for example, Pomi brand
4 tablespoons (36 g) toasted pine nuts, isolated
2 tablespoons (5 g) newly slashed basil
½ teaspoon ocean salt or then again salt, separated
1/8 teaspoon newly ground dark pepper
Run of squashed dried red bean stew chips
2 boneless swordfish filets (¾ pound, or 340 g), set in cooler for 30 minutes for simpler cutting
2 tablespoons (6 g) Fresh Bread Morsels
2 tablespoons (15 g) ground
Pecorino Romano
2 tablespoons (18 g) raisins, doused in warm water for 20 minutes and depleted
1 tablespoon (10 g) finely slashed onion
2 tablespoons (8 g) slashed new, level leaf Italian parsley, isolated
¼ cup (22 g) finely slashed fennel

2 anchovy filets, slashed

METHOD

Warmth 2 tablespoons (30 ml) of olive oil in an enormous skillet over medium warmth. Include the garlic and cook until it discharges its fragrance, 30 to 60 seconds—do not let garlic turn earthy colored.

Mix in the hacked and stressed tomatoes, 2 tablespoons (18 g) pine nuts, basil, ¼ teaspoon salt, pepper, and stew pieces, mix, and spread. Decrease warmth to low and stew for 5 minutes. With a fileting blade, cautiously and perfectly cut the swordfish filets across once into about 1/8-inch (3 mm) thick cuts. Cut each piece to make 4 pieces.

Consolidate the staying 2 tablespoons (30 ml) of olive oil, bread scraps, Pecorino, raisins, remaining pine nuts, staying salt, onion, parsley, fennel, and anchovies in a little bowl, and blend well to consolidate. Recognize the fish pieces on a work surface made sure about with waxed paper or on a tremendous plastic cutting board, and spread 1 tablespoon (12 g) of the bread scrap mix on each piece of fish. Press down solidly with your hands, so the filling sticks.

Cautiously take care of the sides of fish. The sides must be immovably taken care of so that the filling doesn't get away. Beginning at the wide end, move up the fish, totally encasing the filling. Use toothpicks or sticks to make sure about the rolls. Gradually expel top from pureed tomatoes and include the folds into stewing sauce. Spread and cook for 15 to 20 minutes, turning once, or until fish is cooked through.

Move the fish to a serving platter, evacuate sticks, and top with the remaining sauce.

TROUT COOKED IN PARCHMENT

Makes 4 Servings

Soggy and delightful, this simple to-clean cooking strategy is well known all over Italy.

FIXINGS

(4 ounces, or 115 g, each) trout filets
3 cloves garlic, finely cleaved
8 new sage leaves, finely cleaved
½ cup (30 g) finely cleaved new parsley
Pizzazz and juice of 1 lemon
extra-virgin olive oil
1 teaspoon foul ocean salt or salt
Newly ground pepper
Lemon wedges

METHOD

Preheat the broiler to 425°F (220°C). Join the garlic, sage, parsley, lemon pizzazz and juice, olive oil, salt, and pepper in a little bowl. Cut four bits of material paper—every more than twofold the size of the trout. Spot 1 trout on each bit of material and similarly appropriate ¼ of garlic herb blend on each fish.

Brush any residual garlic herb blend over the fish and overlap the material over the fish. Overlay and pleat the edges to seal firmly and place in a preparing dish. Prepare around 10 minutes, until fish is cooked through. Expel from the stove, and present with lemon wedges, permitting visitors to open their own singular bundles at the table.

TURKISH EGGPLAANT AND HERBED RICE PILAF

Makes 4 Servings

Pilafs are accepted to have started in Focal Asia centuries back

FIXINGS

1 pound (455 g) eggplant, cut into
1-inch (2.5 cm) 3D shapes
1/3 cup (80 ml) great quality olive oil, separated
1 huge onion, finely slashed
3 tablespoons (27 g) pine nuts or on the other hand whitened almonds
2 medium ready tomatoes, stripped or, slashed
1 teaspoon grungy ocean salt or salt
Newly ground dark pepper
1 teaspoon unadulterated cinnamon
½ teaspoon allspice
2 tablespoons (8 g) hacked new parsley
2 tablespoons (8 g) hacked new dill
1½ cups (355 ml) Vegetable or
Chicken Stock or water
1 cup (185 g) white basmati rice

METHOD

Preheat the grill. Spot the eggplant on a heating sheet fixed with aluminum foil. Pour ¼ cup (60 ml) of olive oil over the top and blend well to coat. Spot the eggplant under the oven and cook until light brilliant and delicate, around 3 minutes, giving close consideration so they don't consume.

Expel from the stove and put in a safe spot. Add the staying olive oil to a huge pan with a fitting top. Include the onion and sauté 3 to 5 minutes, or until translucent. Mix in the nuts and sauté just until they change shading.

Include the tomatoes, salt, pepper, cinnamon, allspice, parsley, dill, and held eggplant. Mix in stock or water and increment warmth to high. Bring to a bubble. Add the rice to the blend and mix. Lessen warmth to low.

Spot two paper towels over the highest point of the pan. Spread, and stew for 20 to 30 minutes, or until rice is delicate and stock has been retained. Taste, alter seasonings if fundamental, and move to a warmed serving platter

WHOLE WHEAT ORECCHIETE PASTA WITH BROCCOLI AND GARLIC

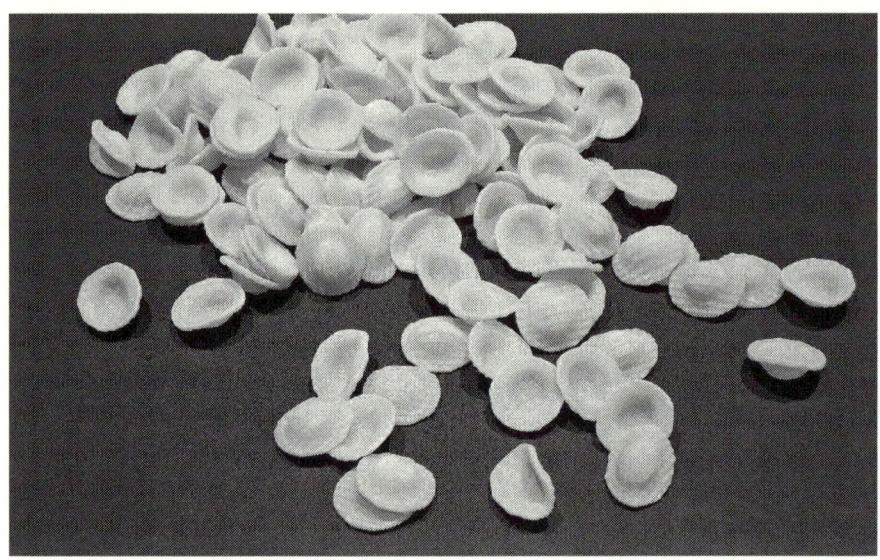

Makes 6 Servings

FIXINGS

1/3 cup (80 ml) great quality, cold pressed olive oil, ideally Puglian
3 cloves garlic, finely hacked
½ chile pepper, minced, or
½ teaspoon squashed red stew chips
¼ cup (35 g) pine nuts
12 little cherry tomatoes, quartered
½ teaspoon grungy ocean salt or salt
¼ teaspoon new ground dark pepper
½ pound (225 g) broccoli florets

2 tablespoons (5 g) newly hacked basil or Italian parsley
1 pound (455 g) entire wheat orecchiette, or any short rice pasta
¼ cup (30 g) ground Pecorino Romano cheddar, for serving

METHOD

Warm the olive oil in a huge, wide skillet over medium warmth. Include the garlic also, chile pepper and sauté around 1 moment, just until they discharge their smell. Include the pine nuts and sauté until softly brilliant. Include the cherry tomatoes, salt, and pepper.

Mix, and cook for 2 minutes. Include the broccoli florets, basil or parsley, and ½ cup (120 ml) water, mix, also, spread. Cook until the broccoli is fork-delicate, 10 to 15 minutes. In the interim cook the pasta in an enormous pot of somewhat salted bubbling water for around 12 minutes, or until still somewhat firm. Channel, and add to the wrapped up sauce.

Hurl to consolidate. Taste and alter seasonings, if essential.

Top with Pecorino Romano cheddar.

SPANISH PAELLA WITH SAFFRON RICE, SHRIMP AND CHICKEN

Makes 8 Servings

FIXINGS

12 medium shrimp
7 hard-shelled mollusks
½ pound garlic-prepared smoked pork wiener
2 pounds boneless chicken
Run of newly ground pepper
¾ teaspoon garlic salt
½ cup extra-virgin olive oil
¼ pound lean boneless pork, cut into ½-inch 3D shapes
½ cup cleaved onion
½ medium red chime pepper, seeded and cut
½ medium yellow chime pepper, seeded and cut
1 huge tomato, stripped and finely slashed
2 cloves new garlic, squashed
3 cups in length grain rice
½ teaspoon salt
¼ teaspoon ground saffron
6 cups water
1 cup solidified peas, altogether defrosted

METHOD

Steam shrimp in a limited quantity of water until simply

pink, at that point set side. Clean mollusks under running water, at that point steam in simply enough water to cover them. When mollusks open, expel from water with an opened spoon and put in a safe spot.

Prick frankfurter with fork in a few spots, place in overwhelming skillet, and spread with cold water. Heat water to the point of boiling and lessen warmth to low. Stew hotdogs, revealed, for 15 minutes. Channel frankfurters well, cut into ¼-inch round pieces, and put in a safe spot. Flush chicken, pat dry, and season with pepper and garlic salt.

In a huge skillet, heat ¼ cup olive oil, include chicken pieces, and fry until brilliant earthy colored. Evacuate cooked chicken from skillet and spot on plate fixed with paper towels. Include wiener pieces to skillet, rapidly earthy colored them, and afterward channel on plate fixed with paper towels.

Expel olive oil from skillet and dry skillet with paper towels. In a similar skillet, heat ¼ cup new olive oil until hot. Include pork blocks and earthy colored rapidly. Include onion, red and yellow ringer peppers, tomato, and garlic.

Cook vegetables and meat, blending continually, until delicate. Put in a safe spot. In an enormous pot, include rice, salt, saffron, and 6 cups of water; heat to the point of boiling and spread, blending periodically, until rice is delicate.

Move rice, shrimp and staying fluid, shellfishes, frankfurter, chicken and pork solid shapes, and vegetables to a broiler safe meal dish. Sprinkle peas over blend, place dish on base rack of a 400degree stove, and prepare for 25–30 minutes or until fluid is assimilated.

Try not to mix. At the point when paella is cooked, expel from broiler, spread with clean kitchen towel, and let represent 5 minutes.

Serve right away.

Note: Broiler ought to be preheated 30 minutes prior paella is put inside.

MEDITERRANEAN ROASTED LAMB AND VEGETABLES

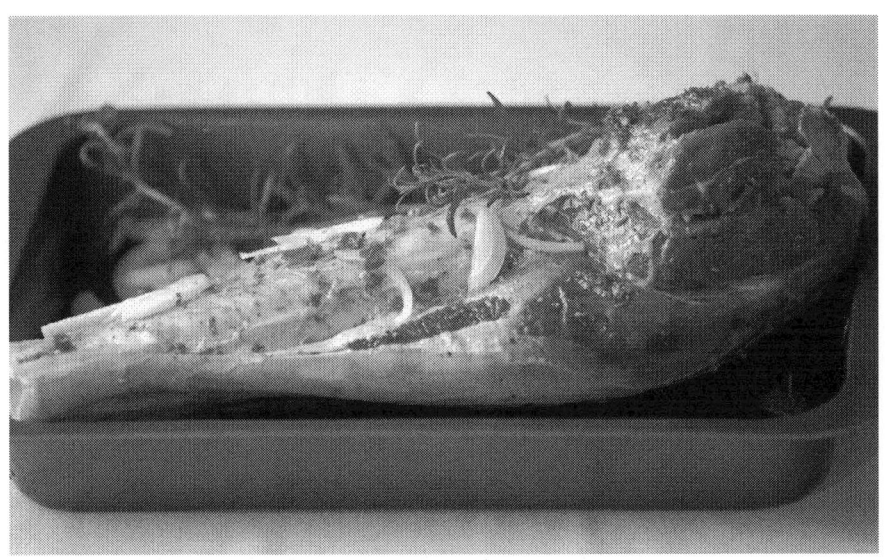

Makes 4 Servings

FIXINGS

Juice from 2 lemons
⅓ cup extra-virgin olive oil
1 clove new garlic, minced
1 tablespoon slashed mint
Salt and newly ground pepper to taste
1½ pounds sheep sirloin, cut into 1½-inch solid shapes
8 enormous inlet leaves
8 new mushroom tops
8 little cherry tomatoes
1 enormous green chime pepper, seeded and cut into 1½-

inch strips
2 little zucchini, cut into 1-inch solid shapes
4 medium onions, quartered
Combine lemon juice, olive oil, garlic, mint, and salt and pepper to taste,

METHOD

Pour over sheep blocks in a resealable plastic baggie. Spot in cooler and marinate for the time being or for in any event 8 hours. On 8 level bladed oiled sticks interchange meat, cove leaves, and vegetables.

Barbecue over hot coals for around 15 minutes, turning sticks a few times. This dish works out in a good way for a slashed serving of mixed greens of onions, cucumbers, tomatoes, and parsley.

Use lemon juice for dressing.

Approx. 296 calories for each serving 38g protein, 8g absolute fat, 3g immersed fat, 0 trans fat, 15g starches, 103mg cholesterol, 141mg sodium, 3g fiber

PREPARED STUFFED TROUT

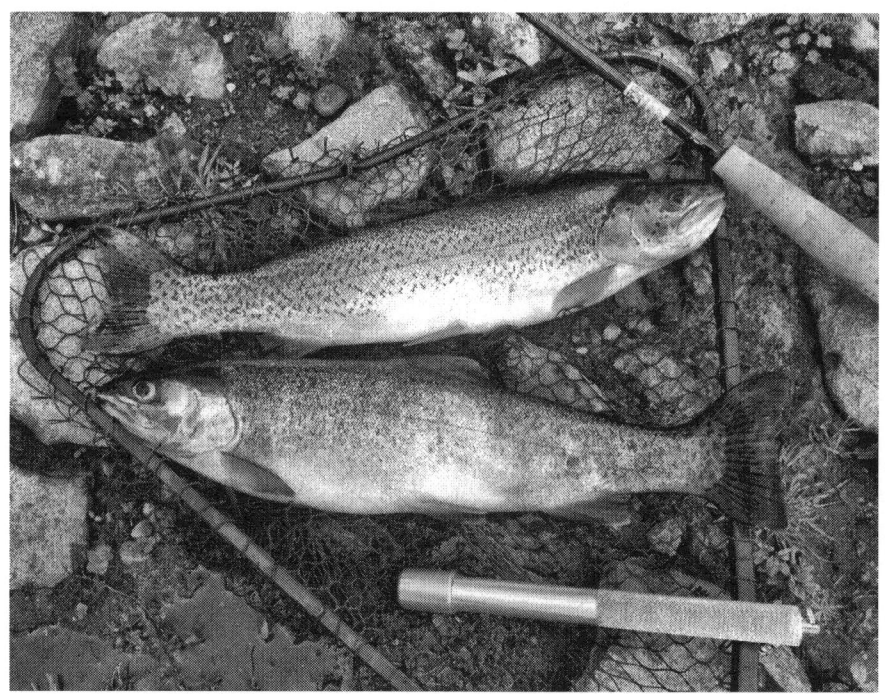

Makes 4 Servings

FIXINGS

3 tablespoons extra-virgin olive oil
1 huge onion, finely slashed
4 cloves new garlic, minced
⅔ cup plain bread pieces
1 lemon, squeezed and skin ground
⅓ cup seedless dull raisins, slashed
½ cup pine nuts
2 tablespoons hacked new parsley

1 tablespoon hacked new dill
Salt and newly ground pepper to taste
¼ cup egg substitute
4 (12-ounce) entire trout, scaled and gutted
Olive oil cooking shower
Lemon wedges for decorate

METHOD

Heat 2 tablespoons of olive oil, include onion and garlic, and cook until delicate, at that point expel from heat. In an enormous bowl, blend bread pieces, ground lemon skin, raisins, pine nuts, parsley, dill, and salt and pepper; include garlic blend and egg and combine well. Stuff every trout with blend and spot in a solitary layer on an oil splashed shallow preparing dish.

Make a few inclining cuts along the body of each fish and sprinkle with lemon squeeze and remaining tablespoon of oil. Prepare at 375 degrees for around 30–45 minutes or until fish drops. Serve hot, embellished with lemon wedges.

NORTHERN BEANS AND CHICKEN

Makes 6 Servings

FIXINGS

2 (3-ounce) skinless, boneless chicken legs
2 (4-ounce) skinless, boneless chicken bosoms
2 onions, slashed into huge pieces
5 carrots, 1 cut and others cut into enormous pieces
2 stems celery, 1 cut and other cut into enormous pieces
Olive oil cooking shower
2 cups canned low-sodium, sans fat chicken stock
4 cups canned Extraordinary Northern beans, depleted and washed
2 tomatoes, stripped and slashed into huge pieces
½ green ringer pepper, hacked into huge pieces
2 teaspoons new thyme
3 cloves new garlic, slashed
2 tablespoons slashed new parsley
Salt and newly ground pepper to taste

METHOD

Flush chicken submerged and pat dry. Spot chicken, half of the onions, 1 cut carrot, and 1 cut celery stem in a pot. Add water to cover chicken, what's more, cook over medium warmth until chicken is delicate. Strain and put in a safe spot. Daintily splash base and sides of a huge meal dish with cooking shower, and include chicken, 2 cups of stock, and beans. Include remaining carrot and celery pieces to meal alongside tomatoes, remaining onion, green chime pepper, thyme, garlic, parsley, and salt and pepper. Prepare for 45 minutes, until blend stews. Serve while hot.

BOUILLABAISSE

Makes 4 Servings

FIXINGS

2 teaspoons extra-virgin olive oil
2 leeks, white and green parts, meagerly cut
3 cloves new garlic, minced
2 cups newly slashed tomatoes
¼ cup dry white wine
1 tablespoon tomato glue
1 tablespoon newly slashed parsley
½ teaspoon dried thyme
2 cove leaves
⅓ teaspoon squashed saffron
⅛ teaspoon fennel seeds
10 ounces new firm cod, cut into 1½-inch lumps
2 (6-ounce) new lobster tails, quartered
16 littleneck shellfishes, cleaned
3 ounces orzo, cooked and depleted

METHOD

In an enormous pan over medium-high warmth, consolidate olive oil, leeks, and garlic; cook for around 3 minutes, blending once in a while. Include tomatoes, 1½ cups of water, wine, tomato glue, parsley, thyme, inlet leaves, saffron, and fennel seeds; mix to consolidate.

Warmth mix to the point of bubbling, blending now and again. Include cod, lobster, also, mollusks; come back to bubble. Lessen warmth to low and stew, secured, for 6–8 minutes. Fish and lobster ought to be cooked until done and mollusks until they open. Expel straight leaves. Spoon cooked orzo into 4 soup bowls; scoop Bouillabaisse over orzo and serve.

BROCCOLI RABE WITH PENNE PASTA

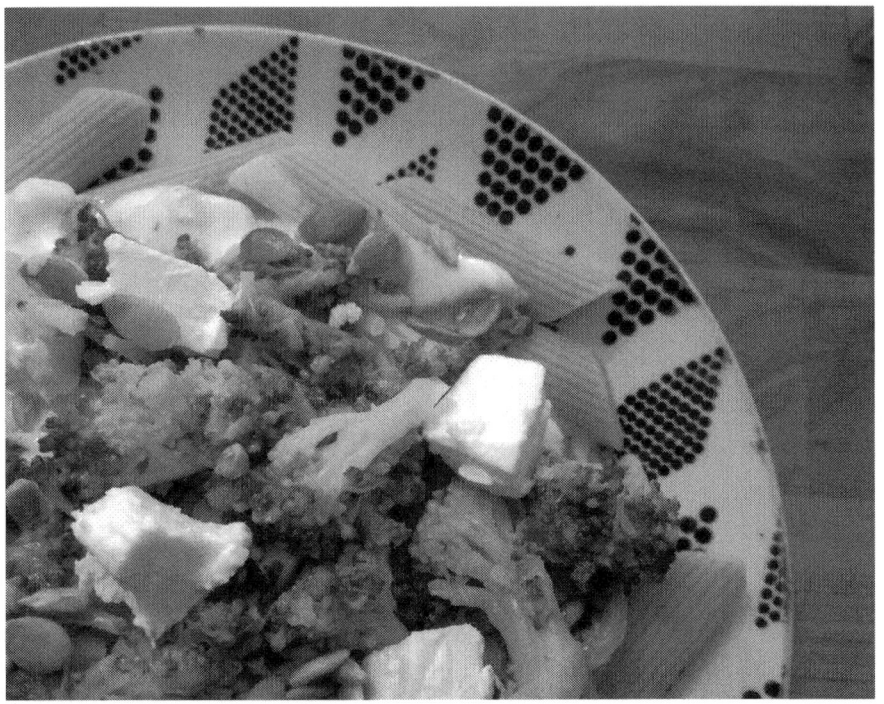

Makes 4 Servings

FIXINGS

2 pounds new broccoli rabe, cleaned, cut, and cut into 1-inch pieces
1 pound entire wheat penne pasta
3 tablespoons extra-virgin olive oil
5 cloves new garlic, meagerly cut
1 medium white onion, slashed
2 ounces anchovy filets, depleted
¼ teaspoon squashed intensely hot pepper chips

Salt and newly ground pepper to taste
Newly ground Romano cheddar for decorate (discretionary)

METHOD

In an enormous pan, heat water and salt to the point of boiling. Include broccoli rabe and cook around 5 minutes, until stems are delicate. With an opened spoon, move broccoli to a colander to deplete. Return broccoli water to a bubble and include pasta. Cook until delicate and channel, holding ¼ cup of pasta water.

Return pasta to a pan and keep warm. In an enormous skillet, heat olive oil, at that point include garlic and onion; sauté for around 2 minutes, until brilliant. Include anchovies and hot pepper pieces, blending for around 1 moment.

Include broccoli rabe and cook an additional 5 minutes, until warmed. To broccoli rabe blend, include pasta and enough of held pasta fluid to softly saturate; hurl until very much blended. Add salt and pepper to taste. Enhancement with Romano cheddar.

Serve warm.

BARBECUED CITRUS SALMON WITH GARLIC GREENS

Makes 4 Servings

FIXINGS

¼ cup orange jelly
2 tablespoons new lime juice
2 tablespoons new lemon juice
¼ cup low-sodium soy sauce
3 teaspoons ground orange skin
4 (3-ounce) salmon filets
2 teaspoons extra-virgin olive oil
2 teaspoons minced new garlic
2 (10-ounce) sacks new spinach
Meager measure of olive oil to rub on fish
Salt and newly ground pepper to taste
1 teaspoon new garlic, crushed to rub on fish
1 piling tablespoon tricks, depleted
1 tablespoon balsamic vinegar
4 scallions, white and light green parts, daintily cut (2–3-inch lengths)

METHOD

Whisk together jelly, lime and lemon juices, soy sauce, and orange skin; pour blend over filets and marinate for 30 minutes in cooler. Get ready barbecue or preheat oven.

Warmth olive oil in a skillet; include garlic and spinach, each pack in turn, and sauté, blending frequently, until spinach is shriveled (around 2 minutes).
Decrease warmth to extremely low, to keep warm. Consolidate olive oil, salt and pepper with crushed garlic. Combine olive oil, salt and pepper with mashed garlicand capers. Rub mixture into both sides of salmon steaks.

Grill the fish orbroil 3–4 inches from flame for 2–2 ½ minutes on each side. Set fish aside.Remove spinach from heat and toss with vinegar; divide equally on 4plates. Add grilled salmon fillet to bed of spinach on each plate andgarnish with scallions. Serve

HOT SHRIMP WITH BLESSED MESSANGER HAIR PASTA

Makes 4 Servings

FIXINGS

8 ounces blessed messenger hair pasta
1½ pounds medium shrimp, stripped and deveined
1 teaspoon low-calorie heating sugar
¼ teaspoon salt
1 tablespoon bean stew powder
½ teaspoon ground cumin
½ teaspoon ground coriander
½ teaspoon dried oregano
1 tablespoon + 1 teaspoon extra-virgin olive oil
Lime wedges for decorate

METHOD

Heat water to the point of boiling. Add pasta, and cook pasta until still somewhat firm. Expel from heat, channel pasta, and come back to pot, sprinkling with sparse measure of olive oil to shield pasta from remaining together.

Put in a safe spot. Sprinkle shrimp with sugar and salt. Join bean stew powder, cumin, coriander, and oregano, at that point gently coat shrimp with zest blend. Warmth 1 tablespoon of olive oil in an enormous nonstick skillet over medium-high warmth.

Include half of the shrimp and sauté around 4 minutes, or until cooked. Expel cooked shrimp from container and rehash methodology with 1 teaspoon olive oil and remaining shrimp. Separation cooked pasta into 4 servings, top with shrimp and skillet sauce, and trimming with lime wedges.

Serve right away.

NATURAL PRODUCT COATED SALMON WITH COUSCOUS

Makes 4 Servings

FIXINGS
¾ pound couscous
2 cups canned low-sodium, sans fat chicken stock, warmed
½ cup apricot jam
3 tablespoons meagerly cut scallion
2 tablespoons arranged horseradish
1 tablespoon white wine vinegar
½ teaspoon salt (partitioned)

4 (6-ounce) salmon filets, 1-inch thick, cleaned
¼ teaspoon newly ground pepper
2 teaspoons extra-virgin olive oil

METHOD

Oil a broiler safe dish and spot couscous in dish. Pour in chicken stock and let sit for 10 minutes until couscous is delicate and fluid is ingested.

Spread dish what's more, keep warm in a low-temperature broiler until prepared to serve. In the interim, join apricot jam, scallion, horseradish, vinegar, and ¼ teaspoon of salt, and mix well with a whisk. Sprinkle salmon filets with staying salt and pepper.

Warmth olive oil in a huge nonstick skillet over medium-high warmth. Include salmon and cook for 3 minutes. Turn salmon and brush with half of apricot blend.

Wrap skillet handle with thwart and prepare salmon in skillet at 350 degrees for 5 minutes or until fish chips. Expel from stove and brush salmon with outstanding apricot blend.

Serve each filet with couscous.

PASTA PRIMAVERA WITH SHRIMP

Makes 4 Servings

FIXINGS

1 pound entire wheat penne pasta
½ cup canned low-sodium, without fat chicken stock
Extra-virgin olive oil to shower + 2 teaspoons
2 dozen medium shrimp, cleaned, stripped, and deveined
1½ cups broccoli florets
1 medium red chime pepper, daintily cut
1 cup split catch mushrooms
1 cup solidified peas
½ cup cut scallions
4 cloves new garlic, minced
1 ounce (2 tablespoons) dry white wine
2 tablespoons newly ground Parmesan cheddar

METHOD

Heat water to the point of boiling. Add pasta, and cook pasta until still somewhat firm. Expel from heat, channel pasta, and come back to pot, showering with sparse measure of olive oil to shield pasta from remaining together.

Put in a safe spot. In an enormous nonstick skillet, heat ¼ cup stock, 2 teaspoons of olive oil, and shrimp; cook until shrimp are pink. With an opened spoon evacuate shrimp and put in a safe spot.

To skillet include remaining ¼ cup of stock, broccoli, red chime pepper, mushrooms, peas, scallions, and garlic. Cook, mixing habitually, for 4–5 minutes, until vegetables are delicate and fluid is for the most part consumed.

Mix in wine, stew about brief longer, and include shrimp to vegetable blend. Spot penne pasta in a huge serving bowl and hurl with staying olive oil. Include vegetable blend; hurl to blend well.

Sprinkle with Parmesan cheddar.

WHOLE WHEAT SPAGHETTI WITH ANCHOVY AND GARLIC SAUCE

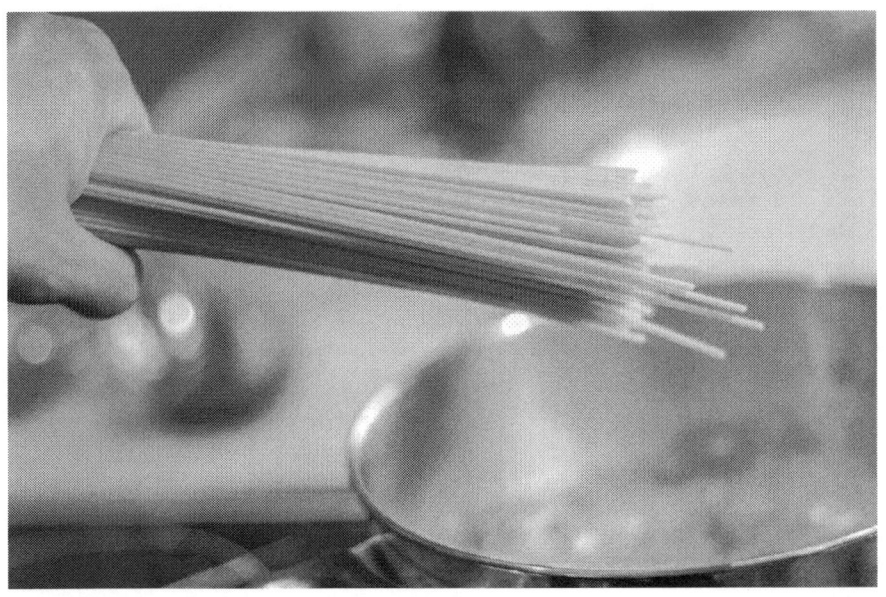

Makes 6–8 Servings

FIXINGS

1 pound entire wheat spaghetti
6 tablespoons extra-virgin olive oil + oil from anchovies
6 huge cloves new garlic, squeezed
2-ounce tin of anchovy filets pressed in oil,
depleted and cleaved Squashed red hot pepper pieces to taste
6–8 pitted dark olives, cleaved
2 tablespoons finely cleaved new parsley
Newly ground pepper to taste

METHOD

Heat water to the point of boiling. Add pasta, and cook pasta until still somewhat firm. Expel from heat, channel pasta, and come back to pot, sprinkling with inadequate measure of olive oil to shield pasta from staying together. Put in a safe spot. Join the two oils and garlic in a skillet over medium warmth and cook around 1–2 minutes.

Include anchovies, breaking into little pieces and mixing to mix well with different fixings. Cook around 30 seconds and expel from heat. Overlay in hot pepper chips, olives, and parsley.

Spot pasta in a huge serving bowl, include anchovy sauce, and hurl to blend. Include pepper to taste, sprinkle with a limited quantity of ground Romano cheddar, if wanted, and serve.

FETTUCCINE WITH SUNDRIED TOMATOES AND GOAT CHEDDAR

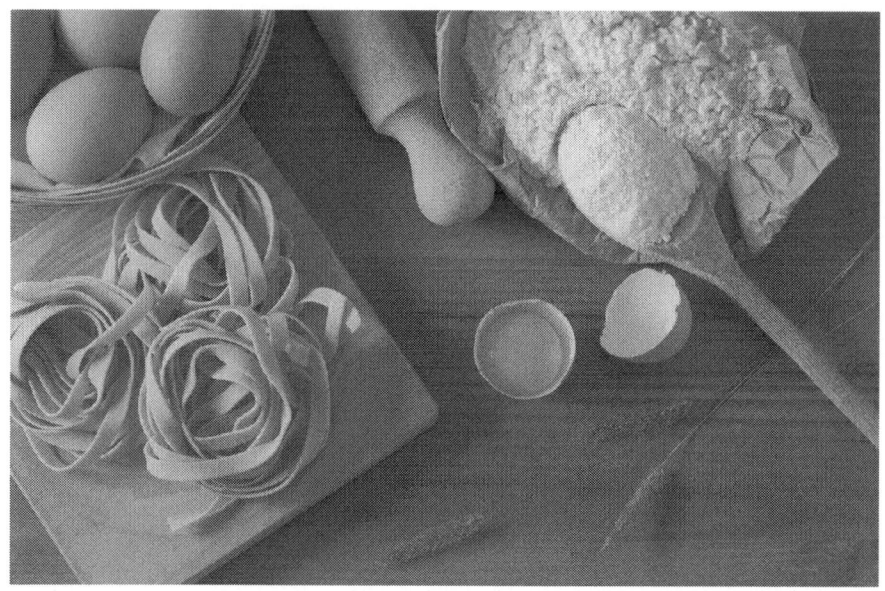

Makes 6–8 Servings

FIXINGS

4 tablespoons cleaved sundried tomatoes (in olive oil)
1 cup cut scallions
4 cloves new garlic, minced
1 medium red ringer pepper, daintily cut
½ cup dry vermouth
¼ cup cleaved new basil
10 pitted Kalamata olives
1 tablespoon escapades, washed and depleted
2 teaspoons dried oregano

1 pound entire wheat fettuccine, cooked and depleted
6 ounces disintegrated low-fat goat cheddar

METHOD

Channel oil from tomatoes and hold oil; put tomatoes in a safe spot. In an enormous skillet, heat oil from tomatoes over medium warmth. Add scallions and garlic to oil and sauté until delicate.

Include red ringer pepper and ¼ cup of vermouth to garlic blend. Cook peppers until fresh delicate or until vermouth is nearly vanished. Diminish warmth to stew, and include tomatoes, remaining ¼ cup of vermouth, basil, olives, escapades, and oregano.

Stew, blending frequently to join flavors (around 5–8 minutes), at that point diminish to exceptionally low warmth to keep warm. Cook pasta to wanted consistency (still somewhat firm would be ideal) and channel. Spot pasta in a huge bowl and hurl with goat cheddar until all around mixed.

Include tomato blend and hurl once more until all around blended. Serve.

FLORENTINE BROILED PORK

Makes 6–8 Servings

FIXINGS

4 pounds lean flank pork
4 cloves new garlic, cut flimsy
½ teaspoon dried rosemary
4 cloves new garlic, entirety
5–6 tablespoons water
6–8 tablespoons generous red wine (don't utilize a cooking wine)
Salt and newly ground pepper to taste

METHOD

On the off chance that the skin of the flank has not as of now been scored, cut lines into skin about ⅛ inch separated. Slice through the tissue deep down on one side and supplement the garlic cuts and rosemary.

Press the entire garlic cloves into the scored skin of the midsection also, place flank into a simmering dish in a 350-degree stove with water and wine.

Sprinkle midsection liberally with salt and pepper and meal for 2–2½ hours or until meat is exceptionally delicate yet soggy, seasoning once in a while.

Present with an assortment of your preferred vegetables.

CHICKEN WITH POMEGRANATE SAUCE

Makes 6–8 Servings

FIXINGS

4 pounds skinless, boneless chicken bosom, cut into little pieces
2 teaspoons paprika
Salt and newly ground pepper to taste
¼ cup extra-virgin olive oil
4 cloves new garlic, minced
2 medium yellow onions, hacked
¼ cup hacked new parsley
1 little hot banana pepper, finely hacked
3 tablespoons Thick Pomegranate Molasses
3–4 cups canned thick tomatoes, undrained

METHOD

Wash chicken, evacuate fat, and cut into little pieces. Sprinkle with paprika furthermore, salt and pepper.

Warmth olive oil in a pot, include chicken pieces, and sautéed food for around 2–3 minutes.

Include garlic and sautéed food for another 2–3 minutes. Include onions, parsley, hot banana pepper, Thick Pomegranate Molasses, and tomatoes with fluid; cover and bring to bubble.

Cook over medium-low warmth for around 30 minutes until chicken is delicate. Present with rice.

CHICKEN PICCATA

Makes 4 Servings

FIXINGS

4 (3-ounce) skinless, boneless chicken bosom filets, gently beat
Salt and newly ground pepper to taste (discretionary)
2 teaspoons extra-virgin olive oil, partitioned
3 cloves new garlic, minced
1 cup canned low-sodium, sans fat chicken stock
2 tablespoons dry white wine
4 teaspoons lemon juice
1 tablespoon universally handy flour

2 tablespoons cleaved new parsley
1 tablespoon escapades
Lemon wedges for decorate

METHOD

Flush chicken bosom filets under virus water and pat dry, at that point place bosoms between layers of wax paper and delicately pound filets with a meat hammer. Gently sprinkle each filet with salt and pepper, whenever wanted.

Warmth 1 teaspoon of olive oil in a huge substantial skillet over medium warmth, include chicken filets, and cook until filets are delicately sautéed and focuses cooked (juice will run clear). Move filets to a serving platter and put in a low-temperature broiler to keep warm. Include remaining teaspoon of olive oil and garlic to same skillet and cook for 30 seconds to relax.

Consolidate chicken stock, wine, lemon squeeze, and flour in skillet. Mix to mix and keep blending until blend thickens. Include parsley and escapades to sauce. Expel chicken from stove, place each filet on a plate, and spoon blend over filets.

Embellishment with lemon wedges. Present with cooked spinach linguine or pasta of decision

PASTA FRESCA WITH CRAB AND LEMON

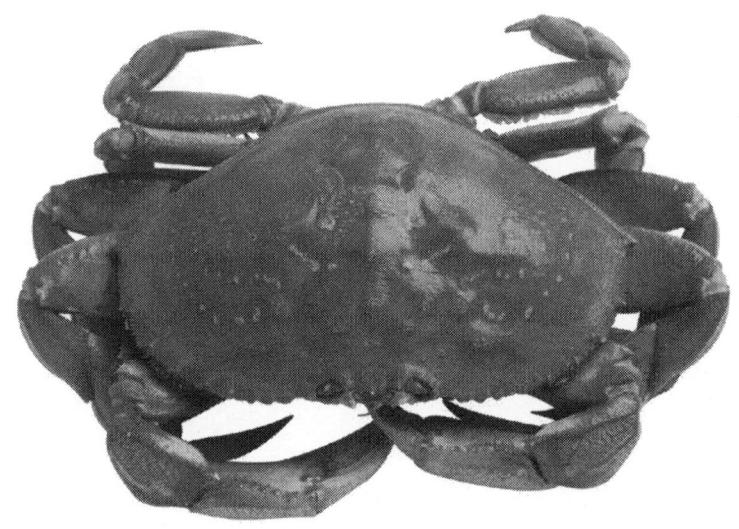

Makes 2 Servings

FIXINGS

5 tablespoons olive oil, partitioned
2 cloves new garlic, minced
1 cup grape tomatoes, divided
1 red jalapeño pepper, seeded and meagerly cut
Salt to taste
2 tablespoons cleaved new basil + more for embellish
1 tablespoon trans fat–free canola/olive oil spread
1 little shallot, finely cleaved
10 ounces cooked and shelled kind sized protuberance crabmeat

4 tablespoons white wine or vermouth
1 (9-ounce) bundle of new linguine pasta
½ of a new lemon to crush
Finely ground Parmesan cheddar for decorate

METHOD

In an enormous skillet, heat 4 tablespoons of olive oil over medium-high warmth. Include garlic and sauté until fragrant and begins to sizzle. Include tomatoes and cook for a few moments until they start to separate.

Diminish warmth to a stew and include jalapeño cuts, salt, and 2 tablespoons cleaved basil. Mix blend and cook for an additional 2 minutes. Move tomato blend to a little bowl and put in a safe spot.

In the same skillet, heat canola/olive oil spread with staying olive oil over medium high heat. Include shallot and sauté until softly carmelized. Include crabmeat, delicately sautéing until crabmeat starts to brown. Add wine to crab blend, delicately scratching free bits of crabmeat and different bits from sides and base of skillet.

Return held tomato blend to crabmeat blend and delicately mix to join, lessening warmth to extremely low to keep sauce warm. Cook new pasta according to bundle guidelines and channel. Add pasta to tomato blend and hurl to cover.

Gap pasta into 2 parts and top with remaining cleaved basil. Press new lemon juice over each serving and sprinkle with Parmesan cheddar.

Serve right away.

SALMON WITH SHRIVELED SPINACH

Makes 4 Servings

FIXINGS

½ tablespoon earthy colored sugar
½ tablespoon smoked paprika
½ teaspoon Saigon cinnamon
½ teaspoon orange get-up-and-go
¼ teaspoon salt or to taste
(4-ounce) salmon filets, skinless
2 teaspoons olive oil
3 teaspoons new minced garlic
1 (9-ounce) sack new spinach

METHOD

Preheat stove and a shallow substantial bottomed broiling

skillet to 400 degrees. In a little bowl, consolidate sugar, paprika, cinnamon, orange pizzazz, and salt. Rub both sides of filets equally with zest blend and spot filets on roaster.

Broil for approximately 10 minutes, turning once after around 5 minutes or until fish drops without any problem with a fork. While fish is broiling, add olive oil to a skillet over medium warmth, at that point include garlic and sauté until fragrant.

Include a couple of lots of spinach at once, until everything is shriveled. At the point when filets are cooked, separate spinach onto 4 plates, top each with a salmon filet, and serve.

STUFFED ZUCCHINI WITH VEGETABLES AND SWEET ITALIAN

Makes 6 Servings

FIXINGS

6 enormous zucchini squash
2 tablespoons olive oil + more to sprinkle
Salt and newly ground pepper to taste

2 cups torn stale bread, outside layer expelled
2 cups sans fat milk
2 cloves new garlic, minced
1 little onion, finely slashed
1 yellow ringer pepper, finely minced
½ pound ground turkey frankfurter
½ cup ground Parmesan cheddar
1 teaspoon dry Italian flavoring blend
2 tablespoons cleaved new parsley

METHOD

Preheat broiler to 375 degrees. Cut zucchini. With a melon spoon, scoop out the zucchini substance to shape a cavity. Hold fragile living creature and put in a safe spot.

Remove a cut from the base of every zucchini piece to permit squash to lie level in the base of a goulash dish. Sprinkle each piece with olive oil, season with salt and pepper to taste, and put in a safe spot. Spot the torn bread in a bowl and include milk.

Permit bread to mellow in fluid for 10 minutes. Warmth 2 tablespoons olive oil in an enormous skillet over medium-high heat. Include garlic, onion, and yellow ringer pepper and sauté until delicate.

Include held cleaved zucchini fragile living creature and keep on cooking until delicate, around 5 minutes. In an enormous bowl, consolidate hotdog, sautéed vegetables, Parmesan cheddar, Italian flavoring, and parsley. Crush milk from bread and add bread to blend. Utilizing your hands, blend fixings to mix.

Stuff the cavity of every zucchini with a liberal measure of stuffing blend. Spot goulash dish with stuffed zucchini on the center rack of broiler and prepare for 20–30 minutes until hotdog is cooked through and carmelized.

MUSTARD SHRIMP

Makes 4 Servings

FIXINGS

1 tablespoon olive oil
2 cloves new garlic, minced
¾ canned cup low-sodium, without fat chicken stock
1 pound crude medium shrimp (around 30–32 shrimp), stripped and deveined
¼ cup new nectar mustard plate of mixed greens dressing, locally acquired
½ teaspoon garlic powder
Salt and newly ground pepper to taste

METHOD

In a huge skillet, heat olive oil and include garlic. Sauté until garlic is delicate. Include stock and shrimp and cook until shrimp gets pink and cooked through. Lessen warmth to low to keep shrimp warm.

In a pan, warm the nectar mustard dressing with garlic powder and salt and pepper. Channel fluid from shrimp and add warmed mustard blend to shrimp, at that point come back to low warmth while mixing to cover shrimp and join flavors, around 5 minutes.

Serve right away.

PEPPERED FILLETS OF SOLE

Makes 4 Servings

FIXINGS

1 tablespoon olive oil
1 tablespoon trans fat–free canola/olive oil spread
2 cups cut catch mushrooms
1 medium shallot, finely slashed

(4-ounce) sole filets
1 teaspoon lemon pepper flavoring
1 teaspoon paprika
Cayenne pepper to taste
1 medium tomato, slashed
2 scallions, meagerly cut

METHOD

In an enormous skillet over medium warmth, dissolve olive oil and canola/olive oil spread. Include mushrooms and shallot and sauté until delicate. Spot filets over mushroom blend.

Sprinkle each filet with lemon pepper flavoring, paprika, and cayenne. Spread skillet and cook over medium warmth until fish drops without any problem. Partition into 4 segments and sprinkle each presenting with tomatoes and scallions.

Serve while hot.

SPICY RAINBOW TROUT

Makes 4 Servings

FIXINGS

For Fish:

4 (6-ounce) filets (about ½-inch thickness)
2 teaspoons olive oil
1 tablespoon zest flavoring (underneath)
2 tablespoons slashed new parsley
1 scallion, slashed
Lemon wedges for decorate

For the Flavoring:

1¼ teaspoons newly ground pepper
2 teaspoons salt or to taste
¼ teaspoon cayenne pepper
1 tablespoon paprika
1 teaspoon bean stew pepper
1 teaspoon dried oregano
1 teaspoon dry mustard

METHOD

Preheat grill. Wash filets under virus water and pat dry. Softly oil filets on the two sides with a treating brush. Make flavoring by consolidating ground pepper, salt, cayenne, paprika, bean stew pepper, oregano, and mustard in a bowl.

Sprinkle the two sides of filets with flavoring and spot skin-side down in an oven container. Spot skillet 4–6 creeps beneath oven and sear filets for 4–5 minutes or until fish drops without any problem. Serve filets sprinkled with parsley, scallion, and lemon wedges.

CHICKEN AND GRAIN WITH VEGETABLES

Makes 4 Servings

FIXINGS

¼ cup newly pressed lemon juice
1 teaspoon olive oil
2 cloves new garlic, minced
½ teaspoon dried oregano
¼ teaspoon dried basil
(4-ounce) skinless, boneless chicken bosoms
1½ cups canned low-sodium, sans fat chicken stock
2 cups snappy grain
1 teaspoon olive oil
1 medium carrot, cleaved

¾ cup cleaved new mushrooms
½ cup cleaved green ringer pepper
¼ cup cleaved onion
Salt and newly ground pepper to taste

METHOD

In an enormous, re-sealable plastic baggie, join the initial 5 fixings. Seal pack what's more, shake well to mix fixings. Include chicken, reseal pack, and hurl again until chicken is very much covered.

Refrigerate to marinate for at any rate 60 minutes. In an enormous pan, heat stock to the point of boiling. Mix in grain. Diminish heat, at that point spread and let stew for 10–12 minutes or until delicate.

Heat olive oil over medium-high warmth. Include carrot, mushrooms, green ringer pepper, onion, and salt and pepper to taste. Sauté until pepper and onion are delicate. Mix vegetables into grain and keep warm.

Preheat grill. Spot marinated chicken on a grill skillet around 4–6 crawls from heat. Sear chicken until juices run clear, around 4–8 minutes or until meat thermometer peruses 170 degrees.

Serve chicken filets over grain blend.

2.6 PIZZAS

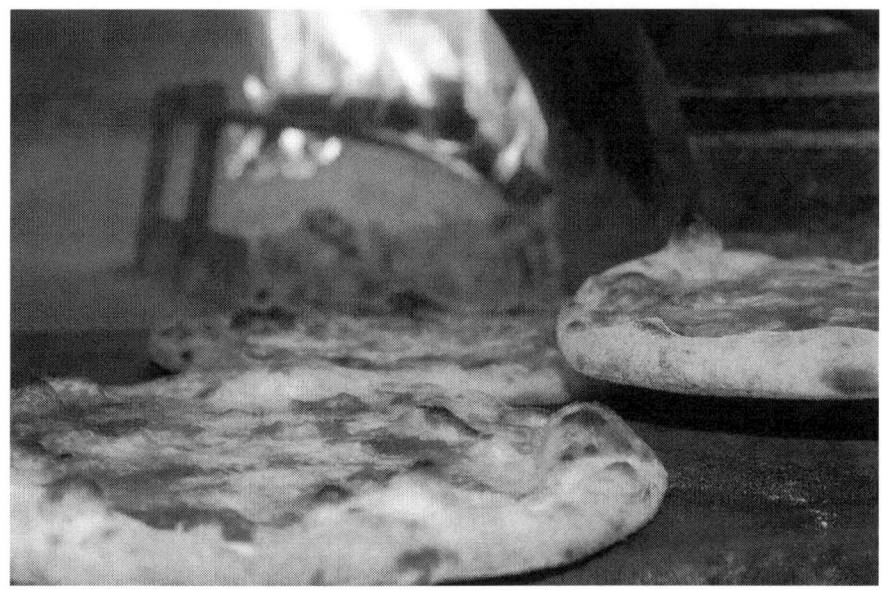

BROCCOLI AND PECORINO FLATBREAD PIZZAS

Makes 4 Servings

FIXINGS

4 oval, trans fat–free entire grain flatbreads
30 new broccoli florets, meagerly cut
2 tablespoons olive oil
3 cloves new garlic, meagerly cut
½ teaspoon squashed super hot pepper pieces or then again to taste
Salt and newly ground pepper to taste

1 cup shaved new Pecorino Romano (around 4 ounces)

METHOD

Preheat stove to 400 degrees. Spot flatbreads on 2 rimmed preparing sheets. In a bowl, hurl together broccoli, olive oil, garlic, hot pepper pieces, and salt and pepper to taste. Dissipate broccoli blend uniformly on flatbreads and sprinkle with Pecorino shavings. Prepare at 400 degrees until flatbreads are fresh and broccoli is searing, around 15 minutes. Serve warm.

MUSHROOM AND SWISS CHEESE PIZZA

Makes an 8-inch pizza

FIXINGS

1 level wrap
1 tablespoon extra-virgin olive oil
½ cup cut arranged mushrooms
2 tablespoons hacked scallions, white and green parts
2 teaspoons new garlic glue
Newly ground pepper to taste
1 ounce destroyed light Swiss cheddar

1 tablespoon dried thyme, finely squashed

METHOD

Preheat stove to 350 degrees. Spot wrap on a preparing sheet and put in a safe spot. Warmth a modest quantity of olive oil in a overwhelming bottomed skillet. Include mushrooms, scallions, garlic glue, and pepper. Sauté for 2–3 minutes, mixing regularly, until mushrooms and scallions mollify.

Expel from warmth and spread blend out uniformly finished wrap. Convey Swiss cheddar over mushroom blend and sprinkle on thyme. Spot in stove and prepare at 350 degrees until cheddar dissolves. Expel from stove and serve.

BASIL AND MOZZARELLA CHEESE PIZZA

Makes an 8-inch Pizza

FIXINGS

1 level wrap
1 teaspoon finely minced new garlic
¼ cup new Traditional Pizza Sauce or a market sauce like Dei Fratelli

¼ cup destroyed part-skim mozzarella cheddar
4 cuts new tomato
4–6 new entire basil leaves

METHOD

Preheat stove to 350 degrees. Spot wrap on a heating sheet. Mix garlic into pizza sauce and spread equally over wrap. Top sauce first with mozzarella cheddar, at that point tomato cuts and basil leaves. Heat at 350 degrees until cheddar liquefies. Expel from stove and serve.

SHRIMP AND MOZZARELLA CHEESE PIZZA

Makes an 8-inch Pizza

FIXINGS

1 level wrap
1 tablespoon new Basil Pesto Sauce (page 488) or a market-new basil pesto
½ cup cooked infant plate of mixed greens shrimp, defrosted (whenever solidified) and all around depleted
4 little hollowed dark olives, depleted and cut
¼ cup destroyed part-skim mozzarella cheddar Dried

chives to sprinkle

METHOD

Preheat broiler to 350 degrees. Spot wrap on a preparing sheet and spread pesto equitably over surface of wrap. Disperse shrimp over pesto, include olives, and top with mozzarella cheddar. Sprinkle chives over cheddar and heat at 350 degrees until cheddar melts and starts to bubble. Expel from broiler and serve.

WHOLE WHEAT PIZZA

Pizza batter goes back to vestige and has establishes in Egypt, Greece, and Rome. Present day pizza (with a tomato besting).

FIXINGS

For the Dough:
1 bundle (¼ ounce, or 7 g) dynamic dry yeast
½ cup (120 ml) tepid water
1½ cups (188 g) entire wheat flour, in addition extra for work surface
1 teaspoon genuine salt

1 tablespoon (15 ml) extra-virgin
olive oil, in addition to extra for bowl

For the Sauce:

1 tablespoon (15 ml) extra-virgin olive oil
1 enormous clove garlic, minced
¾ pound (340 g) stressed (seeded what's more, cleaned) tomatoes, for example, Pomi brand
ocean salt or salt, to taste
Newly ground pepper, to taste
1 tablespoon (2.5 g) finely cleaved
new basil, oregano, or parsley
2 tablespoons (18 g) cornmeal or on the other hand semolina
10 ounces (288 g) new mozzarella cheddar, ground
Ground Parmigiano-Reggiano or on the other hand Pecorino Romano cheddar

METHOD

To make the batter:

Place the yeast in a little bowl and mix in the water. Put in a safe spot. Put the flour into a huge bowl and add the yeast to the middle. Include the salt and olive oil, and mix to consolidate until it frames a thick batter that will be marginally clingy.

On the off chance that the mixture doesn't meet up, include more water, a tablespoon (15 ml) at once. Residue a work surface gently with flour. Massage the mixture vivaciously for 5 to 10 minutes, or until it is smooth and flexible. Shape the mixture into a ball and spot it in a gently oiled bowl. Spread with oiled plastic and a clean kitchen material.

Permit to ascend for 1½ to 2 hours, or until multiplied in size. In the interim, make the sauce.

To prepare the sauce:

Heat the oil in a medium pan over medium heat. Add garlic and decrease warmth to low. At the point when the garlic starts to discharge its smell (before it turns shading), include the tomatoes. Mix and permit the blend to reach boiling point. Include salt, pepper, and new herbs, mix and spread. Lessen warmth to low and stew for 20 to 30 minutes. Permit to cool.

Completing the pizza:

When the mixture has got done with rising, preheat the broiler to 550°F (to 288°C). Punch the mixture down and let it rest 5 minutes. Utilize a turning pin to turn it out into a 10-to 12-inch (26 to 30 cm) measurement circle. Move to a pizza stone or strip cleaned with cornmeal or semolina.

Spread the mixture with a slender layer of sauce, mozzarella, and a sprinkling of Pecorino or Parmigiano cheddar. Crease the edges of the covering in and brush gently with additional olive oil. Prepare on the second-to-least rack for 10 to 15 minutes or until brilliant and bubbly.

Expel from the broiler and permit to stand 5 minutes. Cut and serve.

PIZZA MARGHERITA

Makes a 15-inch pizza

FIXINGS

Meager Crust Pizza Dough 4 Roma tomatoes, daintily cut
Salt and newly ground pepper to taste
½ cup yellow sweet pepper, meagerly cut
¾ cup destroyed part-skim mozzarella cheddar, around 3 ounces
4–5 clipped new basil leaves
¼ cup newly ground Parmesan cheddar
1 tablespoon extra-virgin olive oil

METHOD

Preheat broiler to 450 degrees. Follow bearings for pizza batter and turn out to a 12–15-inch round. Spot mixture on an inadequately oiled pizza container. Spread tomatoes on turned out mixture nearly to the edge of the outside. Sprinkle with salt and pepper to taste.

Top tomatoes with yellow peppers, mozzarella cheddar, basil, and Parmesan cheddar, and sprinkle olive oil over the top. Prepare at 450 degrees for 8– 10 minutes or until covering is fresh and cheeses are softened.

TOMATO, EGGPLANT, AND BASIL PIZZA

Makes an 8-inch Pizza

Fresh Thin Whole Wheat Pizza Dough
1 huge eggplant
6 cloves new garlic, minced
2 tablespoons extra-virgin olive oil
5 medium tomatoes, seeded and cleaved
3 tablespoons cleaved new basil
Spot of squashed super hot pepper drops
3 cups disintegrated non-fat feta cheddar

Salt and newly ground pepper to taste

⅓ cup newly ground Parmesan cheddar for embellish Fresh rosemary, finely cleaved (discretionary)

METHOD

Preheat broiler to 425 degrees. Follow bearings for pizza mixture and turn out to a 12–15-inch round. Spot pizza round on meagerly oiled pizza container.

Cut eggplant down the middle the long way, slicing down the center however not through the skin. Spot on separate dish and heat for 20–30 minutes. Skin ought to be wilted and eggplant delicate.

Evacuate to a plate and hold; when cooled, cut across into slender cuts. In a skillet, sauté garlic in 1 tablespoon of olive oil over low warmth until mollified. Include tomatoes, basil, and hot pepper chips.

Brush pizza batter softly with ½ teaspoon olive oil, top with tomato blend, at that point feta cheddar, and orchestrate eggplant cuts in a pinwheel design, somewhat covering the cuts. Season pizza with salt and pepper also, shower staying olive oil over eggplant. Heat at 425 degrees for 10– 15 minutes until pizza hull is fresh.

Embellishment top of pizza with Parmesan cheddar and rosemary, whenever wanted.

SWEET PEPPER PIZZA

Makes a 15-inch Pizza

METHOD

Entire Wheat Pizza Dough
1 tablespoon extra-virgin olive oil
3 enormous red chime peppers, seeded and daintily cut
3 huge yellow ringer peppers, seeded and meagerly cut
2 cloves new garlic, minced
1 tablespoon slashed new thyme
Salt and newly ground pepper to taste
Crushed intensely hot pepper pieces to taste
1 cup destroyed part-skim mozzarella cheddar

METHOD

Preheat broiler to 500 degrees. Follow headings for pizza batter and turn out to 12–15-inch round. Spot mixture on inadequately oiled pizza dish. Warmth olive oil in substantial bottomed dish furthermore, sauté the red and yellow chime peppers and garlic, around 10 minutes until delicate.

Mix in thyme, salt and pepper to taste, and hot pepper drops. Spread pepper blend over pizza mixture, sprinkle mozzarella cheddar over pepper blend, and prepare at 500 degrees for 20–25 minutes until outside layer is fresh and cheddar has liquefied.

WILD MUSHROOM PIZZA

Makes a 15-inch Pizza

Crust Pizza Dough

3 ounces dried porcine mushrooms
1 quart warm water
2 tablespoons extra-virgin olive oil
4 cloves new garlic, finely minced
1 cup new catch mushrooms, cleaned and daintily cut
1 cup new shiitake or other wild mushrooms
4 tablespoons white wine
1 tablespoon low-sodium soy sauce
½ teaspoon dried thyme
½ teaspoon dried rosemary
Salt and newly ground pepper to taste
3 tablespoons hacked new parsley
8 ounces destroyed smoked provolone cheddar

METHOD

Preheat stove to 425 degrees. Follow bearings for pizza mixture; when prepared, turn it out to a 15-inch round. Spot on insufficiently oiled pizza container. Absorb the dried mushrooms warm water for 30 minutes. Subsequent to dousing, crush overabundance fluid from mushrooms and slash coarsely.

Strain dousing water through a cheesecloth furthermore, put in a safe spot. Warmth 1 tablespoon of olive oil in a heavy bottomed skillet and include half of the garlic. Sauté garlic, blending regularly until it gets brilliant. Include both dried and new mushrooms, sauté for around 5 minutes until they start to discharge their fluid, and afterward include wine and soy sauce.

Keep on sauté until wine vanishes. Add drenching fluid to mushrooms, thyme, rosemary, remaining garlic, and salt and pepper to taste. Increment heat; keep cooking and blending until the majority of the fluid has vanished and mushrooms have gotten coated. Include parsley and expel from heat.

Brush pizza mixture with staying olive oil. Uniformly spread provolone cheddar over outside layer. Spread mushroom blend over cheddar and heat at 425 degrees for about 8–10 minutes, until hull is fresh and cheddar is softened.

SUNDRIED TOMATO AND ANCHOVY PIZZA

Makes a 15-Inch Pizza

FIXINGS

Whole Wheat Pizza Dough

1 red onion, meagerly cut
8 sundried tomatoes in oil, hacked
1 tablespoon new basil leaves, broken in pieces
1 can (2 ounces) anchovy filets, hacked, oil held
1 clove new garlic, minced
1 cup new part-skim mozzarella cheddar,
Salt and newly ground pepper to taste
Finely hacked new parsley for decorate (discretionary)

METHOD

Preheat stove to 425 degrees. Follow headings for pizza mixture; when prepared, roll out to 15-inch round. Spot on meagerly oiled pizza skillet. Top pizza outside layer batter with onion, sundried tomatoes, basil, anchovies, garlic, and mozzarella cheddar. Salt and pepper to taste and prepare at 425 degrees until outside is fresh and cheddar is softened. Enhancement with parsley, whenever wanted.

2.7 DESSERTS, DRINKS AND SMOOTHIES

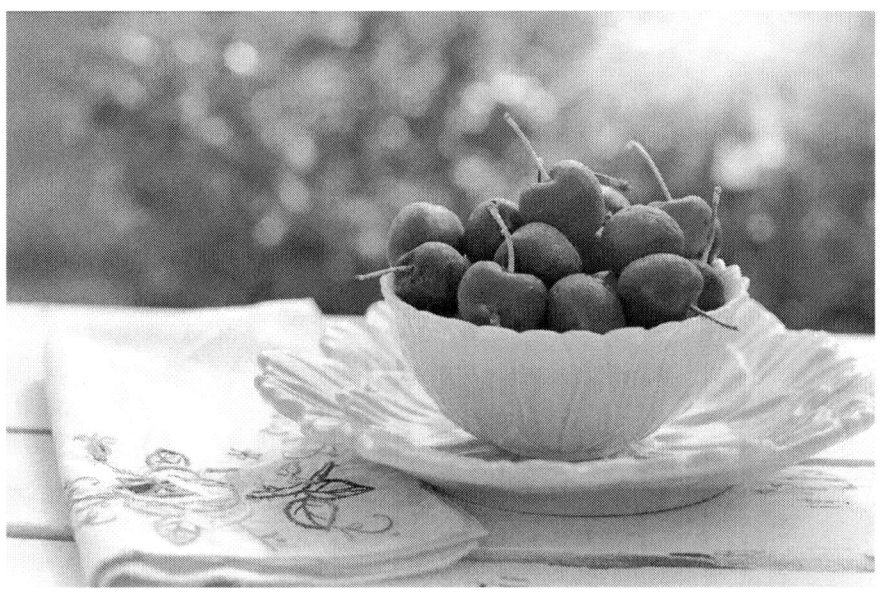

BLUEBERRY BURST WHEY SMOOTHIE

Makes 16 Ounce of Servings

FIXINGS

½ cup cold water
¼ cup new or unsweetened solidified blueberries
2 bundles non-caloric sugar
¼ cup plain non-fat yogurt
1 scoop characteristic seasoned whey protein powder
8 ice 3D squares
Without fat whipped cream

METHOD

Sprinkle of squashed almonds for embellish In an ice-smashing blender, include water, berries, and sugar and mix until smooth. Include yogurt and whey and mix until smooth once more. Include ice 3D squares and hack until squashed. Fill glass. Top with whipped cream and almonds.

SUMMER RHUBARB COOLER

Makes 3 Cups

FIXINGS

¼ cup low-calorie heating sugar
1 cup water
½ pound new rhubarb, cut and cut into 1-inch pieces
1 cup cut new strawberries + extra for decorate
3 tablespoons newly pressed lemon juice

METHOD

3 drinking glasses chilled in cooler. Carry sugar and water

to a bubble in a huge pan over high warmth. Cook, blending frequently, to break down sugar, around 2 minutes.

Decrease warmth to medium and include rhubarb, at that point cook until delicate. Include strawberries and lemon squeeze and cook for 2 extra minutes. Strain blend through a strainer to evacuate solids.

Pour stressed blend into a 9x13-inch preparing dish, spread with saran wrap, and place in cooler. At regular intervals mix blend with tips of fork to separate any framing ice lumps. Freeze blend until slushy and solidified, around 3 hours.

At the point when solidified, scoop into 3 chilled glasses and trimming with staying cut strawberries.

STRAWBERRY PARFAIT WHEY SMOOTHIE

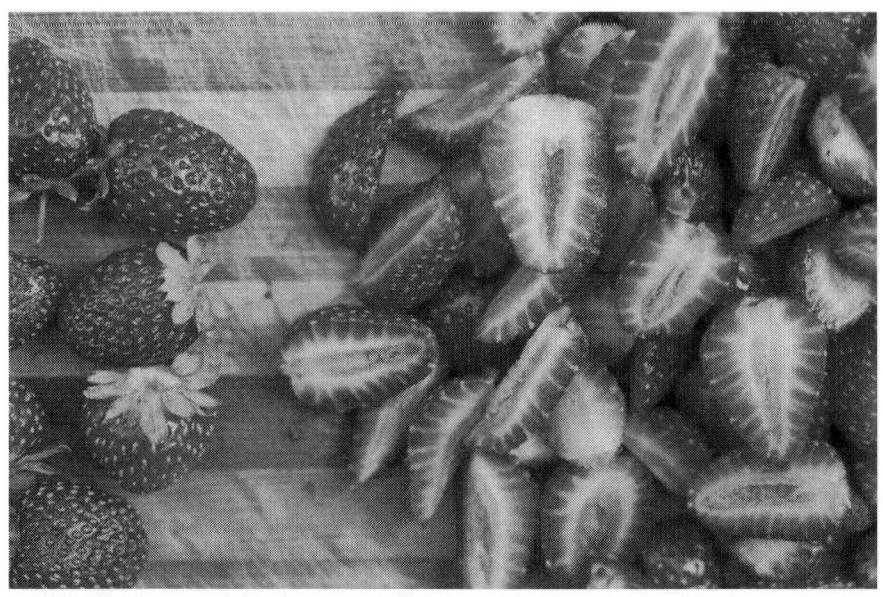

Makes 1 16 ounce Serving

½ cup cold water
½ cup new or unsweetened solidified strawberries
¼ teaspoon vanilla concentrate
2 parcels non-caloric sugar
¼ cup plain non-fat yogurt
1 scoop regular seasoned whey protein powder
8 ice 3D squares
fat whipped cream

METHOD

Without fat, sugar chocolate syrup to sprinkle In an ice-pulverizing blender, include water, strawberries, vanilla concentrate, and sugar, and mix until smooth. Include yogurt and whey, and mix until smooth once more. Include ice and cleave until squashed. Fill glass. Top with whipped cream and chocolate syrup.

CHOCOLATE MOUSSE WHEY SMOOTHIE

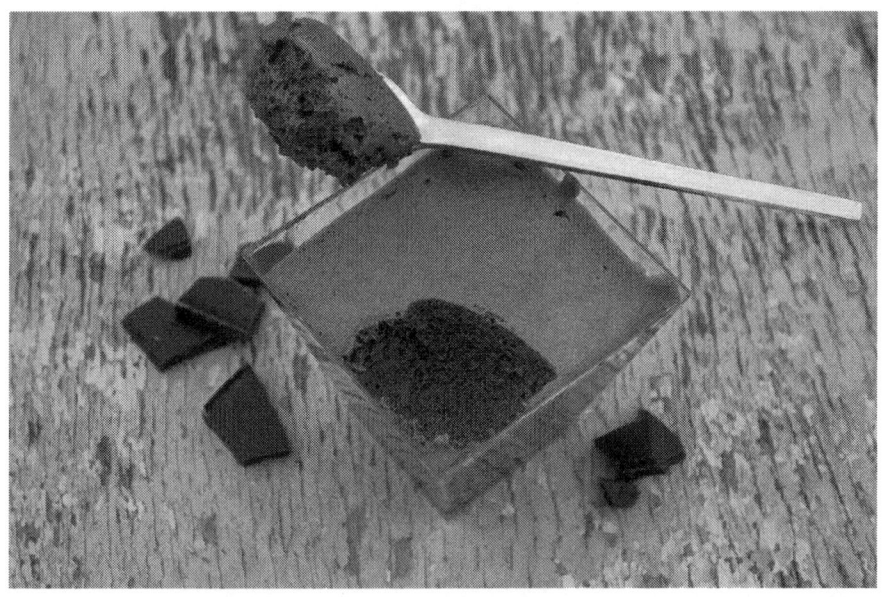

Makes 1 16 ounce Servings

FIXINGS

½ cup cold water

½ cup plain sans fat yogurt
1 scoop regular seasoned whey protein powder
2 bundles non-caloric sugar
1 tablespoon sans fat, without sugar chocolate syrup
1 teaspoon almond extricate
8 ice 3D squares Without fat whipped cream

METHOD

In an ice-pulverizing blender, include water, yogurt, whey, sugar, chocolate syrup, and almond concentrate, and mix until smooth. Include ice and hack until squashed. Fill a glass and top with whipped cream, chocolate syrup, and almonds, whenever wanted.

PINEAPPLE WHEY SMOOTHIE

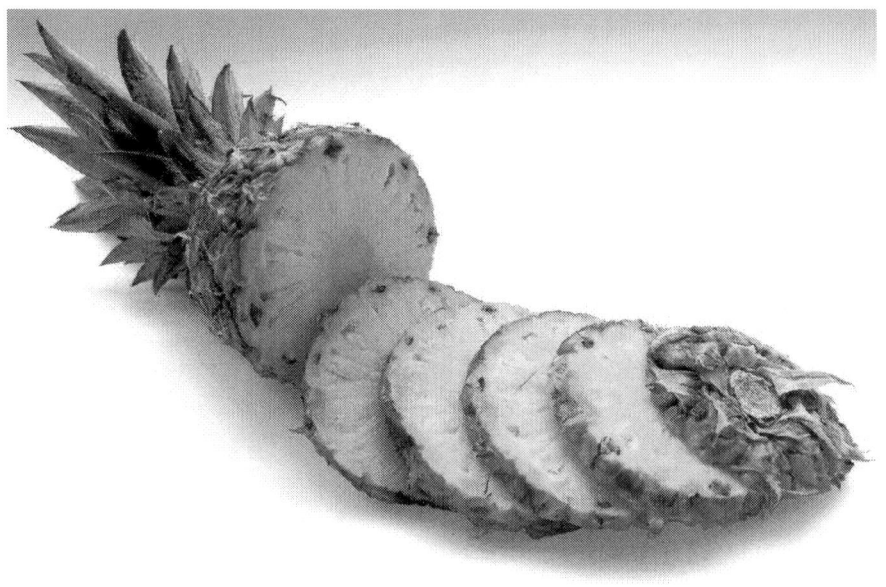

Makes 1 16-Ounce Serving

FIXINGS

½ cup cold water
½ cup new pineapple, diced
1 teaspoon pineapple separate
2 parcels non-caloric sugar
¼ cup plain non-fat yogurt
1 scoop normal seasoned whey protein powder
8 ice solid shapes
fat whipped cream
Squashed pecans for decorate

METHOD

In an ice-squashing blender, include water, pineapple, pineapple remove, and sugar, and mix until smooth. Include yogurt and whey and mix until smooth once more. Include ice and slash until squashed. Fill a glass and top with whipped cream and pecans.

BANANA PEACH VANILLA SOY MILK SMOOTHIE

Makes 1 Smoothie

FIXINGS

1 cup light vanilla soy milk
1 medium banana
1 medium peach, hollowed and cut
1 cup ice
1 teaspoon vanilla concentrate
Non-caloric sugar

METHOD

In a blender join soy milk, banana, peach, and ice. Procedure to wanted consistency; with machine running, include vanilla concentrate and sugar. Serve right away.

CHOCOLATE RASPBERRY SOY MILK SMOOTHIE

Makes 1 16 Smoothie

FIXINGS

1 cup light chocolate soy milk
1 medium banana
1 cup solidified unsweetened raspberries
1 cup ice
1 teaspoon vanilla concentrate
Non-caloric sugar to taste

METHOD

In a blender consolidate soy milk, banana, raspberries, and ice. Procedure to wanted consistency; with machine running, include vanilla concentrate and sugar. Serve right away.

MELON WHEY SMOOTHIE

Makes 1 16-ounce Serving

FIXINGS

½ cup cold water
½ (5–6-inch) new melon
2 bundles non-caloric sugar
¼ cup plain non-fat yogurt
1 scoop characteristic seasoned whey protein powder
8 ice 3D squares
Without fat whipped cream
Squashed almonds for embellish

METHOD

In an ice-smashing blender, include water, melon, sugar, yogurt, and whey, and mix until smooth. Include ice and hack until squashed. Fill glass also, top with whipped cream and almonds.

ORANGE BLOOM PUDDING

Makes 8 Servings

This one make sweet, light, and fulfilling finales to any supper.

FIXINGS

1 pound (455 g) dried apricots
1 cup (200 g) sugar
4 tablespoons (32 g) cornstarch
broken down in ¼ cup (60 ml) cold water
1 tablespoon (15 ml) orange bloom water
Bunch of pistachios, shelled and finely slashed

METHOD

Slash the apricots into little pieces. Spot them in an enormous bowl and spread
them with 4 cups (950 ml) of bubbling water. Spread the bowl with a plate or top. At the point when the apricot pieces separate and about break down, include the sugar, also, mix.

Purée the blend in a blender. Empty the apricot juice into a medium pot. Include the cornstarch blend and mix well with a wooden spoon to consolidate. Set the warmth to high and permit the blend to bubble for 2 minutes, mixing continually.

Diminish warmth to medium-low, include the orange bloom water, and keep cooking the pudding, mixing gradually until it thickens and pulls from the sides of the pot. Fill singular ramekins or a huge embellishing bowl. Sprinkle pistachios on top in an example and refrigerate around 2 hours, or until set. Serve cold.

PEAR AND FIG DESSERT

Makes 4 Servings

This pastry is so rich and delectable that nobody will even understand that it's beneficial for them! Pears are an incredible source of dietary fiber, which brings down cholesterol and forestalls colon disease. Ounce per ounce, figs, one of the world's most seasoned natural products, contain a larger number of supplements than some other organic product.

FIXINGS

4 Bosc pears, stripped
16 dried figs
2 tablespoons (30 ml) lemon juice

2 tablespoons (40 g) nectar
1 teaspoon unadulterated vanilla bean glue or then again unadulterated vanilla concentrate

METHOD

Cut off the bottoms of the pears. Spot the pears furthermore, figs in a medium pan and spread with water. Include the lemon juice, nectar, and vanilla glue.

Heat to the point of boiling over high heat, diminish warmth to medium-low, and stew 20 minutes, or until the pears are delicate. At the point when the pears are sufficiently cool to deal with, expel them from the poaching fluid and stand them upstanding in 4 treat plates.

Shower a couple of tablespoons of cooking fluid over the highest points of the pears furthermore, orchestrate 4 figs around the sides of each plate. Permit to represent 5 minutes at room temperature and serve.

THIN SMOOTHIE

Makes 2 Servings

FIXINGS

½ cup newly crushed tangerine or squeezed orange
½ cup honeydew lumps
½ banana, slashed
1 kiwi, stripped and meagerly hacked
½ cup solidified non-fat plain Greek yogurt or solidified kefir
1 cup infant spinach
¼ cup new mint leaves, in addition to additional branches for embellish

METHOD

Join everything in a blender and mix until smooth and velvety. Serve in two tall glasses and topping with a mint branch.

MANGO SMOOTHIE

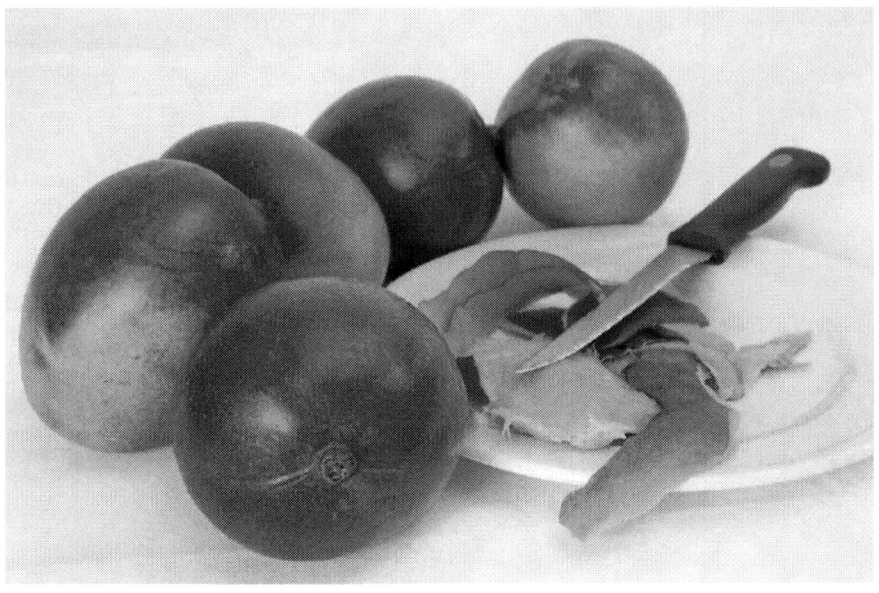

Makes 1 Serving

FIXINGS

1 tbsp. lime juice (newly crushed)
¼ cup nonfat vanilla yogurt
½ cup new mango juice
¼ cup squashed avocado
¼ cup diced mango
½ tbsp. nectar
6 ice solid shapes

METHOD

Join all the fixings in a blender and mix on high until smooth. Pour in a tall serving glass and enhancement with a strawberry or mango cut, if wanted. Appreciate!

PUMPKIN SMOOTHIE

Makes 2 Servings

FIXINGS

½ cup skim milk
½ cup ice, squashed
½ cup pumpkin margarine
⅓ cup of low-fat Greek yogurt
2 tsps. maple syrup
½ tsp. cinnamon
2 tsp. vanilla concentrate

METHOD

Join all fixings in a blender. Mix until smooth. Serve in a glass with a straw.

OAT-BERRY SMOOTHIE

Makes 2 Servings

FIXINGS

½ cup oats
1 cup nonfat arrangement Greek yogurt
1 cup unsweetened almond milk
½ banana
½ cup berries

METHOD

Join all fixings in a blender. Mix until extremely smooth. Appreciate!

BANANA BLUEBERRY BLAST

Makes 2 Servings

FIXINGS

1 ½ cups plain nonfat Greek yogurt
1 cup blueberries
1 banana
5 pecans

½ cup oats

METHOD

Add all the fixings to a blender and mix until extremely smooth. Appreciate!

BERRY BLISS

Makes 2 Servings

FIXINGS

2 cups plain low-fat Greek yogurt
1 tbsp. flaxseed
2 tbsp. almond spread
1 cup solidified blueberries
1 cup solidified strawberries
1 solidified banana

METHOD

Unite all fixings in a blender and blend until smooth

SPINACH CAKE

Makes 12 Portions

FIXINGS

1 ½ pounds spinach, washed
3 tbsp. additional virgin olive oil
1 cup pine nuts
2 cloves garlic, minced
½ cup currants
1 tsp. ocean salt
2 huge eggs, whisked

METHOD

Shrink spinach in a container set over low warmth for around 5 minutes; channel and let cool a piece before pressing dampness out of the spinach. Heartbeat the spinach in a food processor until coarsely cleaved; put in a safe spot.

Warm oil in a skillet; include pine nuts and sauté for a couple of moments or until brilliant earthy colored. Mix in garlic and keep cooking for 1 increasingly minute.

Join the pine nut blend, currants, mixed spinach, eggs and salt in a bowl; spread the blend into a covered heating dish and prepare at 350°F for around 35 minutes.

CITRUS TARTS

Makes 6 Servings

FIXINGS

1 ½ packs solidified smaller than expected phyllo baked good shells
1 cup whipping cream, partitioned
½ tsp. almond remove, partitioned
¼ cup orange curd
¼ cup strawberry curd
New mint leaves for decorate

METHOD

Heat the baked good shells as indicated by the bundle's guidelines and saved until they chill totally. In a food processor, beat ½ cup whipping cream, ¼ teaspoon almond concentrate and orange curd until delicate pinnacles begin to shape.

Spoon this blend into a large portion of the prepared baked good shells. Again beat the staying whipping cream, almond concentrate and strawberry curd in the food processor until delicate pinnacles structure and spoon in the remaining shells.

Trimming with mint leaves and serve.

PISTACHIO AND FRUITS

Makes 12 Servings

FIXINGS

1 ¼ cups unsalted pistachios, broiled
½ cup apricots, dried and hacked
¼ cup dried cranberries
½ tsp. cinnamon
2 tsp. sugar
¼ tsp. allspice
¼ tsp. ground nutmeg

METHOD

Preheat your stove to 350°F and prepare pistachios in a heating plate for around 6 minutes. Put in a safe spot and let them cool totally. Blend all the fixings in a bowl until all around joined and you are prepared to serve.

BRIGTHENED FIGS

Makes 6 Servings

FIXINGS

1 cup dry red wine
½ cup sugar
½ cup balsamic vinegar
1 pound dried figs, expel stems
½ cup mascarpone
¾ cup toasted and cleaved pecans

METHOD

Preheat stove to 350°F and put broiler rack in mid position. Pour the wine, sugar and vinegar in a nonstick pan and heat to the point of boiling over medium warmth, blending continually until the sugar disintegrates.

Add figs to the dish and stew for 5 minutes. Pour the substance of the pot into a clay heating dish and top with pecans. Prepare in preheated broiler for around 30 minutes until the figs assimilate the greater part of the fluid.

Put in a safe spot and let it cool for around 15 minutes at that point present with the sauce and a liberal fixing of mascarpone.

GRAPE DELIGHT

Makes 8 servings

FIXINGS

¾ kg red seedless grapes, washed and depleted
¾ kg green seedless grapes, washed and depleted
¼ cup light cream cheddar, mellowed
⅓ cup low-fat Greek yogurt
1 tsp. vanilla concentrate
2 tbsp. earthy colored sugar
½ cup walnuts, cleaved
¼ cup sugar

METHOD

Split the grapes and put in a safe spot. Join the cream cheddar, yogurt, sugar and vanilla concentrate until well blended. Include the grapes into the blend and fill an enormous serving dish In a different dish, join the earthy colored sugar with the walnuts and utilize this to top the grapes blend totally. Refrigerate for 1 hour, at that point serve.

CITREUS, HONEY CINNAMON

Makes: 4 servings

FIXINGS

4 oranges
2 tbsp. orange blossom water
2 tbsp. crude nectar
1 cinnamon stick
2 ½ tbsp. toasted and cut pecans

METHOD

Strip the oranges and cut them daintily in round shapes. Organize the oranges on a bowl. In the interim, in a little, overwhelming pan, consolidate orange bloom water, nectar and cinnamon stick.

Mix tenderly over low warmth until the blend begins stewing, around 2 minutes. Pour the hot fluid on the oranges and let it cool, at that point top with pecans. Best served when cold.

SWEET CHERRIES

Makes 4 servings

FIXINGS

½ kg new fruits, washed and pitted
2 cups of water
¾ cup sugar
15 peppercorns
1 little vanilla bean, split
3 strips orange get-up-and-go
3 strips lemon get-up-and-go

METHOD

Put fruits in a safe spot. Add rest of fixings to a pot and heat to the point of boiling, blending continually until all the sugar is broken up. Presently, include the fruits and stew for around 10 minutes until delicate however not broken down.

Spill out the froth on a superficial level and put aside to cool. Put in the ice chest for around 2 hours. Strain the fluid before serving. Best delighted in when presented with frozen yogurt.

SUMMER DELIGHT

Makes 3 servings

FIXINGS

⅓ kg peaches, cut
2 tbsp. newly crushed lemon juice
½ jug of sweet red wine
1 tbsp. earthy colored sugar

METHOD

Plunge the peach cuts in lemon to forestall oxidation. Pour the wine in a bowl and add sugar to it, at that point pour in the peaches along with their juice. Spread the bowl and refrigerate for in any event 2 hours. Serve cold.

IMPROVED ROASTED FIGS

Makes 4 servings

FIXINGS

12 ready figs
½ cup sugar
Ricotta cheddar

METHODS

Preheat your broiler to 450°F and mastermind figs on a preparing dish standing upstanding. Then spread sugar on a skillet and spot on low warmth. Shake the skillet to circulate the sugar when it begins liquefying. Keep doing this until all the sugar dissolves, around 15 minutes.

Pour caramel over figs. Presently broil the figs in the caramel for 15 minutes and put aside to cool. Refrigerate the figs for 60 minutes. Orchestrate the figs on plates and shower with the caramel.

Top with the ricotta cheddar.

FIG ICE CREAM

Makes 4 servings

FIXINGS

½ cup ready figs, stems expelled
⅓ cup sugar, in addition to 2 tbsp. sugar
⅓ cup nectar
2 cups cream
1 tsp. anise seed
3 eggs, isolated
1 cup crème fraiche

METHOD

Spot the figs in a food processor and procedure until it frames a puree and move this to a skillet containing ⅓ cup sugar. Cook over medium warmth, blending continually with the goal that it doesn't stick, for around 30 minutes until it shapes such a jam.

In a different pan, heat the nectar, cream, and anise seed and heat to the point of boiling. Mix continually until the nectar disintegrates. Whisk a touch of the hot cream into the egg yolks, empty them into the skillet, and keep blending until the blend thickens and covers the spoon.

Move this to a bowl and pour in the fig blend and crème

fraiche and chill. Whisk the egg whites along with the staying 2 tbsp. sugar until delicate tops structure. Overlay this into the fig blend and put in a frozen yogurt producer, following the directions of the frozen yogurt producer. Serve when prepared.

2.8 SNACKS

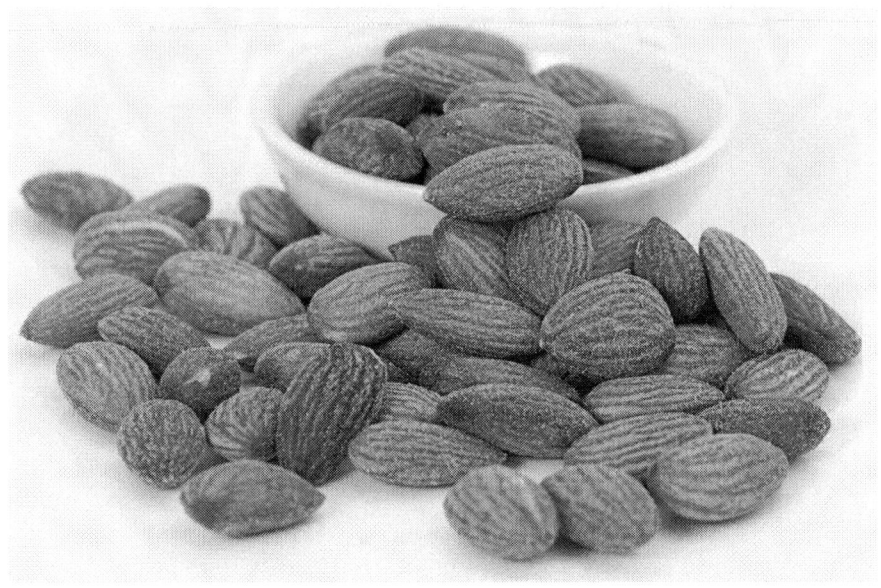

FETA AND GREEK YOUGHURT DIP

Makes 8 servings

FIXINGS

¼ cup disintegrated tomato-basil feta cheddar
2 tbsp. diminished fat mayonnaise
1 (6-oz) holder Greek sans fat plain yogurt
2 tbsp. new parsley, slashed
Grouped new vegetables

METHOD

Combine cheddar, mayonnaise, yogurt and parsley in a little bowl until very much mixed. Partition the plunge among bowls and present with your preferred vegetables.

EGGPLANT AND OLIVE DIP

Makes approximately 2 Cups

FIXINGS

2 (10 ounces every) Italian eggplants, cut into equal parts the long way
1 ½ tsp. additional virgin olive oil, isolated
½ cup pitted green olives, for example, Sicilian or Picholine
½ cup pitted Kalamata olives
Spot of red-pepper chips
1 tsp. finely ground lemon pizzazz
1 garlic clove, meagerly cut
1/4 tsp. coarse salt
1 tsp. new oregano, finely slashed
Little oregano leaves for decorate
Long pizzazz strips for embellish
2 yellow ringer peppers, ribs and seeds expelled, diced

METHOD

Preheat your broiler to 400°F. Mastermind the eggplants, chop side down, on a preparing sheet and brush with ½ teaspoon of additional virgin olive oil. Spread garlic on top and season with ocean salt; cook in the preheated stove for around 20 minutes or until delicate and brilliant. Expel from warmth and let cool for at any rate 5 minutes.

Evacuate and dispose of the eggplant seeds and spoon the tissue into a food processor, alongside garlic; beat until smooth and move to a bowl. Add the olives to the processor and procedure until generally slashed; add to the eggplant blend and mix in the staying additional virgin olive oil, red pepper chips, lemon pizzazz, and the slashed oregano.

Trimming with lemon pizzazz strips and new oregano leaves and present with ringer peppers.

LEMONY GARLIC SESAME HUMUS

Makes Approximately 3 ½ cups

FIXINGS

2 tbsp. toasted white sesame seeds
2 tbsp. additional virgin olive oil
3 stripped and squashed garlic cloves
15 ounces depleted garbanzo beans, fluid saved

2 tbsp. newly pressed lemon juice
2 tbsp. tahini
1 ½ tbsp. minced lemon strip
1 tbsp. minced orange strip
Ocean salt
White pepper

METHOD

Consolidate sesame seeds, additional virgin olive oil, garlic, garbanzo beans (save 1 tablespoon for decorate), lemon juice, and tahini in a food processor; process, including garbanzo bean fluid if fundamental until you accomplish wanted consistency.

Season hummus with ocean salt and pepper and move to a serving bowl. Trimming with the held beans and sprinkle with lemon and orange strip. Refrigerate, firmly secured, until chilled.

Appreciate!

WARM LEMON ROSEMARY OLIVES

Makes 12 servings

FIXINGS

1 tsp. squashed red pepper chips
2 twigs new rosemary
3 cups blended olives
1 tsp. ground lemon strip
1 tsp. olive oil
Lemon turns, discretionary

METHODS

Preheat your stove to 400°F. Spot pepper chips, rosemary, olives and ground lemon strip onto an enormous sheet of foil; shower with oil and overlap the foil. Squeeze the edges of the sheet to firmly seal.

Prepare in the preheated broiler for around 30 minutes. Expel from the sheet and spot the blend to serving dish.

Serve warm decorated with lemon turns.

VELVETY CUCUMBERS

Makes 4 servings

FIXINGS

2 English cucumbers, meagerly cut
1 ½ cups low-fat Greek yogurt
2 tbsp. lemon juice, new
1 ½ tsp. mustard seeds
Coarse salt and ground pepper, to taste
Little bundle dill

METHODS

Join all the fixings in a bowl until all around consolidated.

SIMMERED VEGGIE HUMUS

Makes 20 servings

FIXINGS

1 bulb garlic
¾ cup olive oil, isolated
1 egg plant, divided
1 red ringer pepper, split

⅓ cup lemon juice, newly crushed
2 jars chickpeas, depleted
¼ cup sesame tahini glue
⅓ tsp. smoked paprika
½ tsp. salt

METHOD

Broiler to 450°F and fix a preparing skillet with foil. Cut the extremely top of the garlic bulb off and sprinkle with 1 teaspoon of olive oil. Next envelop it with foil. On a different dish, place the eggplant and chime pepper, sprinkle with 2 tablespoons of olive oil, and hurl so it covers equitably.

Spot the wrapped garlic into the container containing the vegetables. Broil for 30 minutes without covering and cool for 10 minutes. Expel the strips from eggplant and chime pepper and hack the vegetables into little pieces.

Spot the chickpeas in a food processor with a metal cutting edge and procedure until smooth. Next, press the mash from the garlic into the processor; include the various fixings including the broiled vegetables and procedure until all around mixed.

Serve into little serving bowls and serve quickly and refrigerate the leftover portion.

SOUND NACHOS

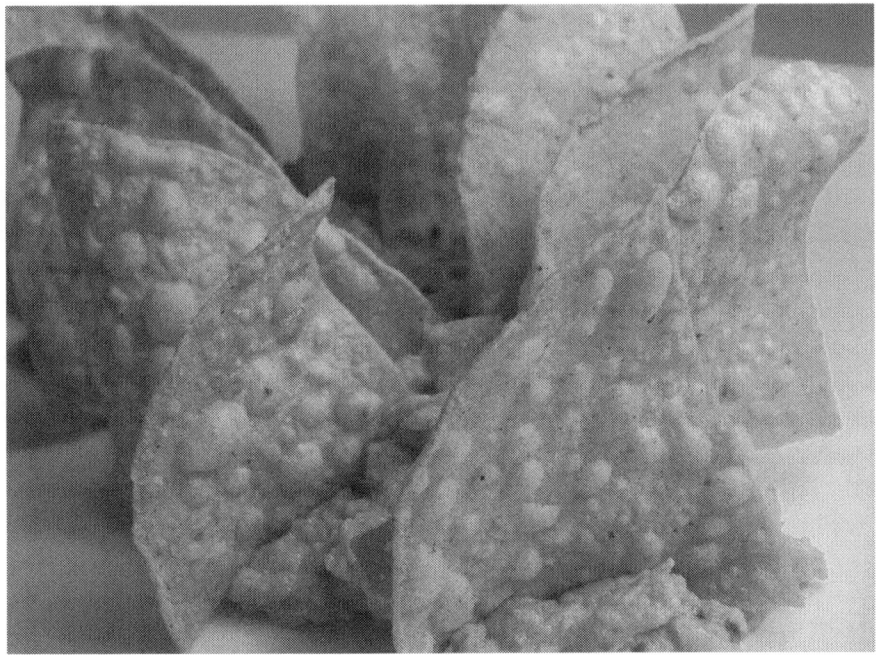

Makes 6 servings

FIXINGS

1 medium green onion, meagerly cut (around 1 tbsp.)
1 finely cleaved and depleted plum tomato
2 tsp. oil from holder of sun-dried tomatoes
2 tbsp. sun-dried tomatoes in oil, finely cleaved
2 tbsp. Kalamata olives, finely cleaved
4 oz. café style corn tortilla chips
1 (4-oz) bundle finely disintegrated feta cheddar

METHOD

Combine onion, plum tomato, oil, sun-dried tomatoes and olives in a little bowl; put in a safe spot. Organize the tortillas chips on a microwavable plate in a solitary layer; uniformly top with cheddar and microwave on high for 1 moment.

Pivot the plate half turn and keep microwaving for 30 additional seconds or until cheddar is bubbly. Uniformly spread the tomato blend over the chips and cheddar and serve.

JALAPENO BOATS

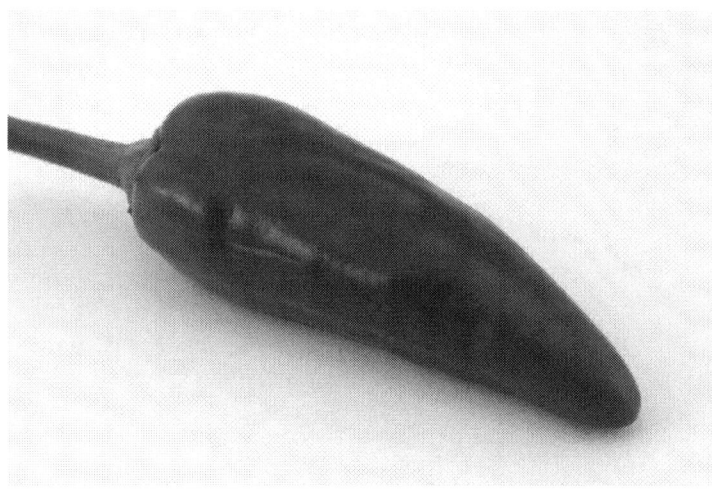

Makes: 44 servings

FIXINGS

1 pack (12 oz.) veggie lover burger disintegrates
1 cup Parmesan cheddar, destroyed
1 bundle (8 oz.) mellowed light cream cheddar
22 enormous jalapeno peppers, cut into equal parts the long way and seeds evacuated

METHOD

Sauté disintegrates in an enormous skillet set over medium warmth for around 5 minutes or on the other hand until warmed through. Join together destroyed Parmesan and mellowed cream cheddar in a little bowl; crease in the disintegrate.

Preheat broiler to 425°F. Spoon around 1 tablespoon of the disintegrate cheddar blend into every jalapeno half; organize the jalapeno parts on a heating sheet, cheddar side up, and heat in preheated broiler for around 20 minutes.

GREEK POTATOES

Makes 4 servings

FIXINGS

¼ cup new lemon juice
2 finely cleaved cloves garlic
1 ½ cups water
⅓ cup olive oil
A touch of ground dark pepper
2 3D shapes chicken bouillon
1 tsp. dried rosemary
1 tsp. dried thyme
6 stripped and quartered potatoes

METHOD

Preheat your stove to 350°F. Combine lemon juice, garlic, water, olive oil, pepper, bouillon 3D shapes, rosemary and thyme in a little bowl. Mastermind the potatoes in a solitary layer in a medium-sized heating dish and top with olive oil blend. Heat secured, turning twice, for around 2 hours or until delicate.

STUFFED CELERY BITES

Makes: 8 servings

FIXINGS

Olive oil cooking shower
1 clove garlic, minced
2 tbsp. pine nuts
8 stems celery
Celery leaves
¼ cup Italian cheddar mix, destroyed
1 (8-ounce) sans fat cream cheddar
2 tbsp. sunflower seeds, dry-simmered

METHOD

Coat a nonstick skillet with olive oil; include garlic and pine nuts furthermore, sauté over medium warmth for around 4 minutes or until the nuts are brilliant earthy colored. Put in a safe spot.

Remove the wide base and tops from celery and expel 2 meager strips from the round side of celery to make a level surface. Consolidate Italian cheddar and cream cheddar in a bowl; spread into celery and cut every celery stem into 2-inch pieces.

Sprinkle half of the celery pieces with sunflower seeds and

half with the pine nut blend; spread and let represent in any event 4 hours before serving.

PESTO-STUFFED MUSHROOMS

Makes 14 servings

FIXINGS

14+ catch mushrooms, washed and stemmed
½ cup additional virgin olive oil
3 cloves garlic
2 cups basil
½ cup pine nuts
1 cup pecans
½ tsp. ocean salt

METHOD

Orchestrate the mushroom tops top-side down on a plate. In a food processor, mix together stuffing fixings until exceptionally smooth. Scoop an equivalent measure of the stuffing into each top and dry out at 105°F until delicate, for around 6 hours. Serve warm.

SQUASH FRIES

Makes 6 servings

FIXINGS

1 medium butternut squash
1 tbsp. additional virgin olive oil
½ tbsp Grapeseed oil?
⅛ tsp. ocean salt

BEARINGS

Strip and expel seeds from the squash; cut into slim cuts and spot them in a bowl. Coat with additional virgin olive oil and grapeseed oil; sprinkle with salt and hurl to cover well. Organize the squash cuts onto three heating sheets and sear in the stove until firm.

COOK BALSMIC BEETS

Makes 4 servings

FIXINGS

3-4 medium beets

2 tbsp. additional virgin olive oil
1 tbsp. balsamic vinegar
½ tsp. ocean salt

METHOD

Scour the beets and wash well; cut into 6 wedges and spot them in a preparing dish. Shower the beets with additional virgin olive oil, vinegar, and salt and heat, secured, at 375°F for around 60 minutes. Reveal and keep heating for 15 additional minutes or until practically delicate.

FIG TAPENADE

Makes 16 servings

FIXINGS

1 cup dried figs
½ cup water
1 cup Kalamata olives
1 tbsp. hacked new thyme
½ tsp. balsamic vinegar
1 tbsp. additional virgin olive oil

METHOD

Heartbeat the figs in a food processor until very much cleaved; include water and keep beating to frame a glue. Include olives and heartbeat until very much mixed. Include thyme, vinegar, and additional virgin olive oil and heartbeat until smooth. Present with pecan wafers.

SOUND SPICED NUTS

Makes 4 servings

FIXINGS

⅔ cup pecans
⅔ cup walnuts
⅔ cup almonds
½ tsp. dark pepper
½ tsp. cumin
1 tsp. stew powder
½ tsp. ocean salt
1 tbsp. additional virgin olive oil

METHOD

Put the nuts in a skillet and toast until delicately seared.

Meanwhile, set up the flavor blend; join dark pepper, cumin, stew powder, and salt in a bowl.

Coat the toasted nuts with additional virgin olive oil and sprinkle with the flavor blend to serve.

COOKED YAM CHIPS

Makes 1 to 2 servings

FIXINGS

1 huge yam
1 tbsp. additional virgin olive oil
Salt

METHOD

Preheat your stove to 300°F. Scour potato and cut into flimsy cuts. Hurl together the potato cuts with salt and additional virgin olive oil in a bowl; organize them in a solitary layer on a treat sheet. Prepare for around 60 minutes, flipping at regular intervals, until firm and cooked.

COOKED ASPARAGUS

Makes 4 servings

FIXINGS

1 pound new asparagus
1 tbsp. additional virgin olive oil
1 medium lemon
1/2 tsp. newly ground nutmeg
1/2 tsp. genuine salt
½ tsp. dark pepper

METHOD

Preheat your stove to 500°F. Organize asparagus on an aluminum foil and sprinkle with additional virgin olive oil; hurl until very much covered. Spread the asparagus in a solitary layer and overlap the edges of foil to make a plate.

Cook the asparagus in the broiler for around 5 minutes; hurl and proceed simmering for 5 minutes more or until cooked. Sprinkle the simmered asparagus with nutmeg, salt, pizzazz and pepper to serve.

2.9 VEGETARIAN MEDITERRANEAN MEALS

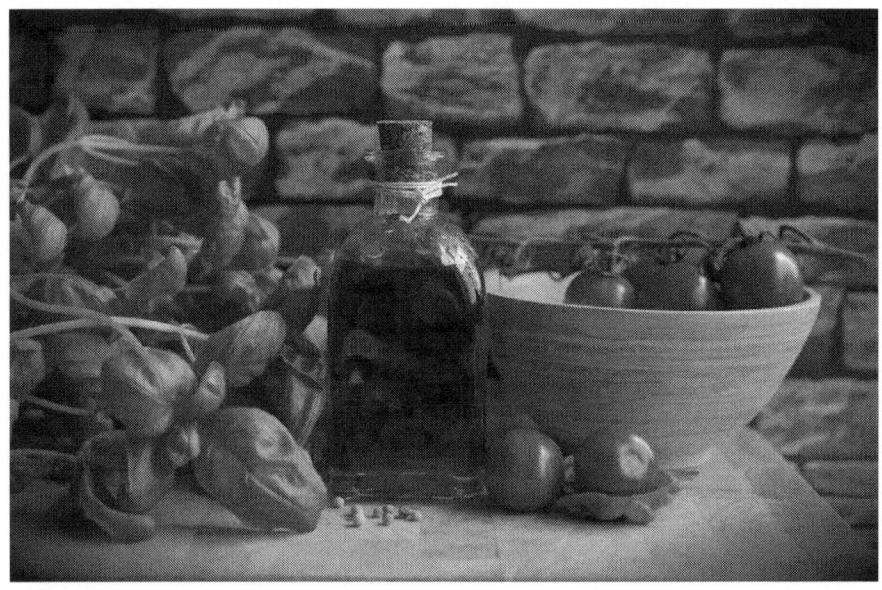

STEWED ARTICHOKES WITH BEANS

Makes 4 servings

FIXINGS

1 ½ pounds fava beans, shelled
3 tbsp. newly pressed lemon juice
4 cups water
24 child artichokes
1 lemon half, to rub artichokes
2 tsp. additional virgin olive oil
4 twigs new level leaf parsley
4 twigs new thyme

1/4 tsp. squashed red-pepper chips
1/4 tsp. newly ground dark pepper
1 tsp. ocean salt
3 stripped and delicately squashed cloves garlic
1 lemon half, to rub artichokes

METHOD

Fill a huge bowl with water and ice; put in a safe spot. Add water to a medium pot and bring to a turning bubble over high warmth. Include fava beans and whiten for around 30 seconds.

Expel the beans from boiling water and add to a bowl with ice shower; let douse for around 5 minutes or until cold. Strip the skin from the fava beans and put in a safe spot.

In an enormous bowl, consolidate lemon juice with 4 cups of water; put in a safe spot. Expel the extreme external leaves from the artichokes and remove the tips. Trim each stem and strip; rub with the lemon half and spot in the lemonwater blend.

Add additional virgin olive oil to a pan set over medium warmth; heat until hot yet, not smoky. Include garlic, red pepper chips, ocean salt and dark pepper; cook, blending, for around 2 minutes or until the shallot is delicately cooked.

Mix in the artichokes, parsley, thyme, and 1 cup of lemon-water blend; carry the blend to a delicate stew. Lower warmth to medium low and keep stewing, secured, for around 14 minutes or until the artichokes are delicate. Include the fava beans and keep cooking for 3 minutes more or until the beans are delicate.

Serve right away.

MEDITTERANEAN PASTA WITH OLIVES, TOMATOES, AND ARTICHOKES

Makes: 4 servings

FIXINGS

12 ounces entire wheat spaghetti
2 tbsp. additional virgin olive oil, isolated
2 garlic cloves, cut
½ medium onion, meagerly cut the long way
Coarse salt and ground pepper
½ cup dry white wine
1 artichoke heart, flushed and cut the long way
1 16 ounces grape or cherry tomatoes, split the long way, isolated
⅓ cup pitted Kalamata olives, cut longwise

½ cup new basil leaves, torn

¼ cup ground Parmesan cheddar, in addition to additional for serving

METHOD

Cook pasta in a huge pot of bubbling salted water following bundle directions, until still somewhat firm; channel and hold 1 cup of pasta water. Return the cooked pasta to the pot.

Meanwhile, heat 1 tablespoon of additional virgin olive oil; include garlic and onion, season with ocean salt and dark pepper and cook, blending normally, for around 4 minutes. Mix in wine and keep cooking for around 2 minutes more or until the fluid is vanished.

Mix in the artichoke and keep cooking for around 3 minutes more or until beginning to brownMix in half of the tomatoes, and olives and cook for 2 minutes. Include pasta and mix in the staying olive oil, tomatoes, basil and cheddar;

Include the held pasta water, as wanted, to cover the pasta. Serve promptly with additional cheddar.

SWISS CHARD WITH OLIVES

Makes 4 servings

FIXINGS

1 ¼ pounds cut and washed Swiss chard
1 tsp. additional virgin olive oil
2 garlic cloves, cut
1 little yellow onion, cut
1 jalapeno pepper, hacked
⅓ cup Kalamata olives (salt water restored), pitted and generally hacked
½ cup water

METHOD

Separate stems from leaves of Swiss chard; cut the stems into little pieces what's more, generally slash the leaves; put in a safe spot. Warmth additional virgin olive oil to a Dutch stove or an enormous skillet over medium heat.

Include garlic, onion, and jalapeno; sauté for around 6 minutes or until onion is delicate and translucent. Include olives, Swiss chard stems, and water and cook, secured, for around 3 minutes.

Mix in the chard leaves and keep cooking, secured, for around 4 minutes or then again until the leaves and stems are delicate. Serve right away.

BARBECUED VEGGIES TANGINE

Makes: 6 servings

FIXINGS

¼ cup brilliant raisins
6 little red potatoes, cut in quarters
¼ cup pine nuts, toasted
2/3 cup couscous, uncooked
2 garlic cloves, squeezed
1 medium red onion, wedged
1 tsp. fennel seeds, squashed
¼ tsp. cinnamon, ground
1 ¾ cups onions, slashed
1 tsp. additional virgin olive oil
1 tsp. cumin, ground
¼ cup green olives, hollowed and slashed
1 ½ cups water
¼ tsp. newly ground dark pepper
Cooking shower
2 red ringer peppers, diced
1 green ringer pepper, diced
½ tsp. fit salt

2 tsp. balsamic vinegar
½ can tomatoes, slashed

METHOD

Set up a gas or charcoal barbecue. Join the ringer peppers, red onion, and ¼ teaspoon ocean salt, vinegar and ½ teaspoon olive oil in a zip lock plastic pack and hurl well.

Spot an enormous nonstick pan on medium warmth and include the remaining olive oil and include the garlic and slashed onion. Sauté these for around 3 minutes and include fennel, cumin and cinnamon.

Let them cook for a further brief at that point include the staying salt, olives, raisins, potatoes, tomatoes, dark pepper and water and carry the container to a bubble. Spread the pot, and stew for 25 minutes or until the potatoes are delicate.

Expel the onions and chime peppers from the plastic sack and barbecue on a rack covered with cooking splash for around 10 minutes. Heat up the rest of the water in a different pot and gradually mix in the couscous.

Expel from warmth and spread the container and let it represent 5 minutes. Serve the tomato blend over couscous and top with the flame broiled onions, chime peppers and pine nuts.

CHIROZO PILAU

Makes: 4 servings

FIXINGS

1 tbsp. additional virgin olive oil
1 huge red onion, daintily cut
¼ kg child cooking chorizo, cut
4 garlic cloves, minced
1 tsp. paprika, smoked
1 can tomatoes, cleaved
¼ kg basmati rice
4 garlic cloves, minced
½ liter stock
1 little pack parsley, cleaved
Get-up-and-go of 1 lemon, stripped in thick strips and the rest of
2 straight leaves, new

METHOD

Spot a thick pot on medium warmth and pour in the oil. Include the onion and let it cook until brilliant earthy colored for around 6 minutes. Push the onions aside of the skillet, pour in the chorizo and let it cook until it begins discharging a portion of its oils.

The garlic and paprika are straightaway. Mix for 2 minutes,

at that point include the tomatoes and let cook for 5 minutes. Pour in the rice, lemon pizzazz, sound leaves and stock. Mix everything in the skillet and heat to the point of boiling.

Spread the skillet and stew for 12 minutes. Turn of the warmth, take the top off and spread the dish with foil, at that point put the top back on and let it sit for around 15 minutes. Mix in the parsley and present with lemon wedges. (Crushing in the lemons gives the dish an astonishing taste.)

PASTA WITH RAISINS GABANZOS AND SPINACH

Makes: 6 servings

FIXINGS

8 ounces farfalle (tie) pasta
2 tbsp. additional virgin olive oil
4 garlic cloves, squashed
½ cup chicken stock (unsalted)
½ (19 ounces) can flushed and depleted garbanzos
4 cups slashed new spinach
½ cup brilliant raisins
2 tbsp. Parmesan cheddar
Split dark peppercorns

METHOD

Fill a pot ¾ full with salted water; bring to a turning bubble over high warmth. Include pasta and cook for around 12 minutes or until still somewhat firm; channel and set aside. Warmth additional virgin olive oil in an enormous skillet and sauté garlic until fragrant; include chicken stock and garbanzo beans and mix until warmed through.

Mix in spinach and raisins and cook for around 3 minutes or until spinach is withered. Partition pasta among plates and top each with around 1/6 of sauce, peppercorns and Parmesan.

Serve immediately.

EGGPLANT STEAK WITH DARK OLIVES, SIMMERED PEPPER AND FETA CHEDDAR

Makes: 4 servings

FIXINGS

Balsamic Marinade
2 cloves garlic, minced

1 tbsp. low-sodium tamari
1 tbsp. balsamic vinegar
¼ tsp. newly ground dark pepper
2 tbsp. additional virgin olive oil
Eggplant Steaks
1 enormous eggplant, around 1 lb.
¼ lb. disintegrated feta cheddar
2 simmered red peppers, diced
1 ½ cups chickpeas, depleted
4 tsp. balsamic vinegar
Spot of oregano
½ cup pitted dark olives
Ocean salt
Newly ground dark pepper
4 (6½-inch round) pita breads
New oregano, for decorate

METHOD

In a bowl, consolidate marinade fixings, bit by bit mixing in additional virgin olive oil until all around joined. Put in a safe spot. Preheat your oven or barbecue. Cut the eggplant into 4 ¼-inch-thick cuts, longwise to look like steaks.

Brush the eggplant cuts with the marinade and sear or barbecue for around minutes per side or until delicate. Move the flame broiled eggplants to the plates, one on each.

In a little bowl, consolidate feta, red peppers, chickpeas, oregano and dark olives; season with ocean salt and ground dark pepper. Mix until all around mixed; mix in some marinade.

Flame broil or toast pita bread and cut into wedges; put in a safe spot. Spoon around 2 scoops of the olive-pepper blend onto eggplant "steak" and shower with balsamic vinegar. Include a couple of pita bread wedges and trimming with oregano branches. Rehash with the rest of the fixings and serve right away

PART 3 – CALORIES TABLE

The calories table is an indispensable tool to keep under control the daily energy supply provided by a diet. In addition to calories, in every table are indicated the amount of protein, carbohydrates and fats provided by each food and the percentage breakdown of calories provided by macronutrients.

To speed up the consultation, only the most frequently used foods in Mediterranian Diet are listed. The values are to be considered indicative, as the nutritional characteristics of the food can vary according to the brand or variety of the food. For particularly variable foods, the table indicates the specific brand to which the values refer.

The values shown in the Carbohydrates, Proteins and Fats columns are the macronutrients (in grams) contained in 100 g of food. The values of the Calories column are the calories (kcal) supplied by 100 g of food.

The last column, % kcal C-P-F, indicates the percentage of calories supplied by the various macronutrients, Carbohydrates-Proteins-Fats. For example, for dried chickpeas, the value 59-24-17, indicates that 59% of total calories are provided by carbohydrates, 24% by proteins and 17% by fats (remember that carbohydrates and proteins provide four calories per gram, while one gram of fat provides 9 calories).

3.1 MAIN FOODS

Food	Carbohydrates	Protein	Fats	Calories	% kcal C-P-F
Fatty meat (beef)	0	16	28	316	0-20-80
Lean meat (veal)	0	21	4	120	0-70-30
Dried chickpeas	47,5	19,5	6,1	323	59-24-17
Classic corn flakes	84	7	1	373	90-8-2
Crackers	77,4	11,6	1,5	370	84-13-4
Rice Crackers	83,1	7,6	1	372	89-8-2
Dried beans	45	23	1,2	283	64-33-4
Flour	74	11	1	349	85-13-3
Corn flour	78	8,1	1,4	357	87-9-4
Dried broad beans	54	22	2	322	67-27-6
Rice breadsticks	83,1	7,6	1	372	89-8-2
Lentils	54	25	2,5	339	64-30-7
Marmelade	47	0,8	0	191	98-2-0
Honey	80	0,8	0	323	99-1-0
Mortadella	1	16,5	29	327	1-20-79
Olive oil	0	0	100	900	0-0-100
Green olives	0,4	1	15	136	35125
Bread	53	7	1,8	256	83-11-6
Pasta	72	12	1,5	350	82-14-4
Fresh pasta	66	15	4,5	365	72-16-11
French Fries	49	4,1	36	536	37-3-60
Degreased raw ham	0	29	5	161	0-72-28
Rice	75	8	1	341	88-9-3
Salmon	0	22	10	178	0-49-51
Durum wheat flour	72,4	12,5	1,7	355	82-14-4
Natural mackerel drained	0	25	7	163	0-61-39
Tuna	0	26	2	122	0-85-15
Eggs	0,5	12,4	8,7	130	2-38-60
Sugar	100	0	0	400	100-0-0

3.2 DAIRY

Food	Carbohydrates	Protein	Fats	Calories	% kcal C-P-F
Butter	0	0	82	738	0-0-100
Charterhouse	2	14,5	24	278	3-21-76
Crescente	2	15	25	293	3-20-77
Milk flakes	2,2	11,9	3,9	92	10-52-38
Grana cheese	0	33	28	384	0-34-66
High quality whole milk	5	3,2	3,7	66	30-19-50
Low-fat milk	4,9	3,1	1,5	46	43-27-30
Lerdammer	0,1	27	28	360	0-30-70
Mozzarella	0,5	20	15	213	1-38-61
Cooking cream	4	3	22	226	07/05/1988
Philadelphia classic	3,1	4,6	28	278	04/07/1989
Fresh ricotta	4	8	13	165	10-19-71
Whole white yogurt	4,9	3,9	4,2	73	27-21-52
Sweetened whole fruit yogurt	14,7	3,2	3,6	104	57-12-31

3.3 FRESH FRUIT

Food	Carbohydrates	Protein	Fats	Calories	% kcal C-P-F
Apricot	7	0,4	0,1	31	92-5-3
Pineapple	10	0,5	0,1	43	93-5-2
Watermelon	3,5	0,3	0,1	16	87-7-6
Orange	7,4	0,6	0,2	34	88-7-5
Banana	14,5	1,1	0,3	65	89-7-4
Persimmon (kaki)	16	0,6	0,2	68	94-4-3
Clementina	12,6	0,8	0,2	55	91-6-3
Cherry	9	1	0,1	41	88-10-2
Date	73	2,2	0,2	303	96-3-1
FIG	10,4	0,9	0,2	47	89-8-4
Strawberry	6	0,7	0,3	30	81-9-9
Kiwi	9,1	1,2	0,5	46	80-11-10
Raspberry	6,2	1	0,6	34	73-12-16
Tangerine	15	0,8	0,2	65	92-5-3
Apple	11	0,3	0,1	46	95-3-2
Melon	8,1	1	0,2	38	85-10-5
Medlar	6,1	0,4	0,4	30	82-5-12
Pear	10	0,4	0,1	43	94-4-2
Fishing	6	0,9	0,2	29	82-12-6
Plum	10	0,5	0,1	43	93-5-2
Grapes	15	0,7	0,2	65	93-4-3

3.3 VEGETABLES

Food	Carbohydrates	Protein	Fats	Calories	% kcal C-P-F
Asparagus	5	5	0,2	42	48-48-4
Beets	5	1	0,1	25	80-16-4
Beets	4	1	0	20	80-20-0
broccoli	5,2	2,8	0,4	36	58-31-10
Artichokes	3	2	0,2	22	55-37-8
carrots	8	1,2	0,2	39	83-12-5
Cauliflower	4,5	5,5	0,3	43	42-52-6
Brussels sprouts	7	6	0,7	58	48-41-11
Cucumbers	3,5	1	0,5	23	62-18-20
Fennel	7	1,2	0,1	34	83-14-3
mushrooms	1,5	3	0,3	21	29-58-13
Lettuce	3,5	1,2	0,2	21	68-23-9
Eggplant	5,7	1	0,2	29	80-14-6
Potatoes	18	2	0,2	82	88-10-2
peppers	6,7	0,9	0,3	33	81-11-8
tomatoes	4	1	0,2	22	73-18-8
Celery	3	1	0,2	18	67-22-10
spinach	4	3	0,3	31	52-39-9
Pumpkin	4	1,1	0,1	21	75-21-4
Zucchini	4	2	0,1	25	64-32-4

Manufactured by Amazon.ca
Bolton, ON